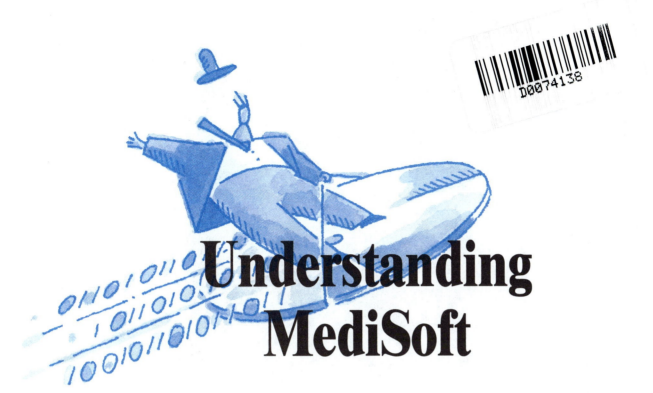

Understanding
MediSoft

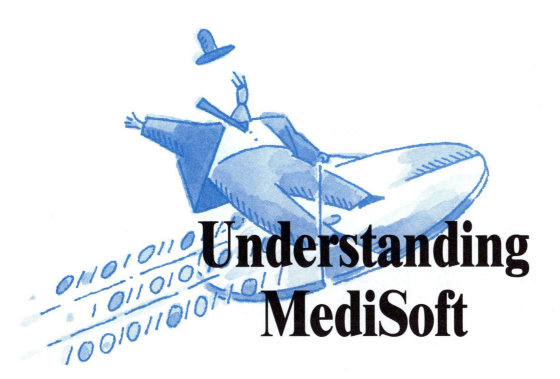

Understanding
MediSoft

A Real Life™ Book
Including a Simulated Work Program

Second Edition

ICDC Publishing, Inc.

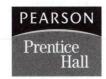

PEARSON

Prentice
Hall

Upper Saddle River, New Jersey 07458

Library of Congress Cataloging-in-Publication Data

Understanding Medisoft : including a simulated work program. -- 3rd ed.
   p. cm. -- (A real life book)
   ISBN-13: 978-0-13-219401-3
   ISBN-10: 0-13-219401-5
 1. MediSoft. 2. Medical fees--Computer programs.

R728.5.U53 2006
610.285--dc22

                                2007045750

Publisher: Julie Levin Alexander
Publisher's Assistant: Regina Bruno
Executive Editor: Joan Gill
Associate Editor: Bronwen Glowacki
Director of Marketing: Karen Allman
Senior Marketing Manager: Harper Coles
Marketing Specialist: Michael Sirinides
Managing Production Editor: Patrick Walsh
Production Liaison: Julie Li
Production Editor: Sarvesh Mehrotra
Media Product Manager: John Jordan
Manager of Media Production: Amy Peltier
New Media Project Manager: Stephen J. Hartner
Manufacturing Manager: Ilene Sanford
Manufacturing Buyer: Pat Brown
Senior Design Coordinator: Maria Guglielmo
Interior Designer: Amy Rosen
Cover Designer: Solid State Graphics
Composition: Aptara, Inc.
Printing and Binding: Edwards Brothers
Cover Printer: Phoenix Color

Credits and acknowledgments borrowed from other sources and reproduced, with permission, in this textbook
appear on appropriate page within text.

Pearson Education Ltd.
Pearson Education Singapore Pte. Ltd.
Pearson Education Canada, Ltd.
Pearson Education—Japan
Pearson Education Australia Pty. Limited

Pearson Education North Asia Ltd.
Pearson Educación de Mexico, S.A. de C.V.
Pearson Education Malaysia Pte. Ltd.
Pearson Education Inc., Upper Saddle River, New Jersey

10 9 8 7 6 5 4 3 2 1
ISBN 13   978-0-13-219401-3
ISBN 10   0-13-219401-5

Disclaimer

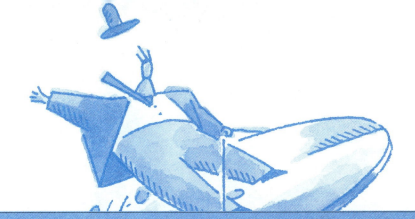

This manual is a guide for learning and practicing the skills of a medical biller. Decisions should not be based solely on information within this manual. Decisions affecting the practice of medical billing and patient accounting must be based on individual circumstances including legal/ethical considerations, local conditions, and payor policies.

The information contained in this manual is based on experience and research. However, in the complex, rapidly changing medical environment, this information may not always prove correct. Data used are widely variable and can change at any time. Billing personnel should follow current coding regulations outlined by official coding organizations.

The publisher and author do not accept responsibility for any adverse outcome from undetected errors, opinion, and analysis contained in this manual that may be inaccurate or incorrect, or from the reader's misunderstanding of an extremely complex topic. All names used in this book are completely fictitious. Any resemblance to persons or companies, current or no longer existing, is purely coincidental.

Acknowledgments

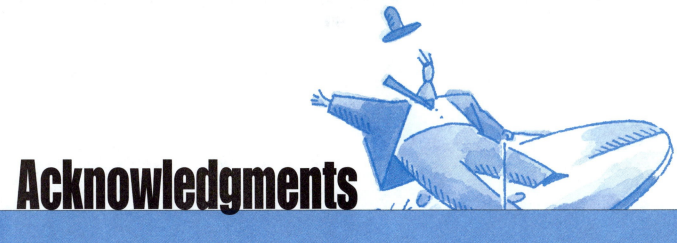

Many people have contributed to the development and success of *Understanding MediSoft*. We extend our thanks and deep appreciation to the many students and classroom instructors who have provided us with helpful suggestions for this edition of the text.

We would like to express our thanks to the following individuals:

Linda Jepson
Janet Grossfeld, Adelante Career Institute, Van Nuys, CA
Hollis Anglin and Michael Coffin, Dawn Training Institute, New Castle, DE
Michael Williams and Tim McCall, 4-D College, Colton, CA
Anna McCracken and Lynn Russell, American Career College, Los Angeles, CA
Jeff Ward, MediSoft/NDC Health, Mesa, AZ
L'Tanya Knight, Institute of Medical Studies, Irvine, CA

Thanks to the CPA firm of Miller, Kaplan, Arase and Company, LLP:

Mannon Kaplan, C.P.A.
George Nadel Rivin, C.P.A.
Joseph C. Cahn, C.P.A.
Edwin Kanemaru, C.P.A.
Kenneth R. Holmer, C.P.A.
Douglas S. Waite, C.P.A.
Charles Schnaid, C.P.A.
Donald G. Garrett, C.P.A.
Catherine C. Gardner, C.P.A.
Jeffrey L. Goss, C.P.A.

And finally to:

Sean Adams
Sydney Adams
Floree Brown
Nathaniel Brown Sr.

Preface

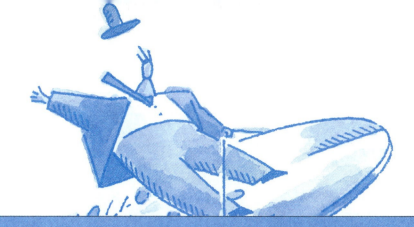

Welcome to the exciting world of medical billing. This book contains instructional training in the Medisoft Patient Accounting computer program, as well as a simulated work program to help you experience the real life situations that a medical biller goes through.

This text is designed to enable you to work through the material at your own pace. In the simulated work portion, the outside margin of this text has been enlarged to allow room for taking notes and jotting down procedure and diagnosis codes.

Features of the 2nd edition include:

- **Based on Medisoft version 12:** Learners can use the student tutorial packaged with this text or request a copy of the networkable software from their sales representative.
- **Screen Shots:** Numerous screen grabs from the Medisoft program make learning visible and easy.
- **Simulated Work Program:** Allows students practice and experience as a medical biller using Medisoft.
- **Exercises and Review Questions:** Build retention and ask students to think critically.

Section 2 includes training using the Medisoft Patient Accounting software system. Medisoft is one of the most comprehensive and popular computerized medical billing software programs available today. The Medisoft Patient Accounting System not only creates claims for billing insurance carriers, but also keeps track of patient accounts and creates most of the forms necessary for running a medical office.

While this book is complete in teaching the Medisoft patient accounting program, it should not be consid-ered a complete text for learning medical billing. It is important that trainees not only learn to enter data into a computer billing program, but also to understand the concepts behind what they are entering. The simulated work portion of this text incorporates concepts that are not taught by simple data entry, for example CPT, ® and ICD-9-CM coding, privacy guidelines, patient record keeping, reception area duties, correspondence, and manual completion of claims.

On occasion you will be asked to enter data contained in a document (i.e., enter the charges shown on Document 4). All documents are contained in Section 4 of this text. Numerous forms used in the medical office are contained in Sections 5 & 6 in the back of this text and may be copied as needed.

Note Regarding Dates:

Please note that when YY is used in reference to a date the YY indicates the current year (12/01/YY). When PY is used in reference to a date the PY indicates the prior year (or last year) (12/01/PY). When NY is used in reference to a date NY indicates the next year (12/01/NY).

Note Regarding Birth Dates:

When a birth date is referenced with CCYY- ## this indicates to subtract the ## from the current year to determine the birth year. Example: 10/04/CCYY-14 (using the year 2006 for the CCYY) = 2006 -14 = 1992; therefore, the birth date would be 10/04/1992.

GOOD LUCK as you venture into a challenging, but fulfilling career.

Contents

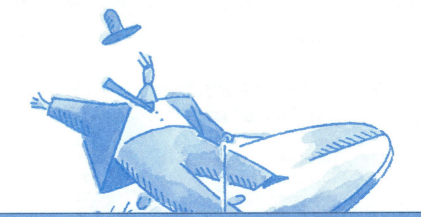

SECTION 5

Petty Cash and Window Payments 185

SECTION 6

Patient File Forms 199

Appendix A 205

Appendix B 217

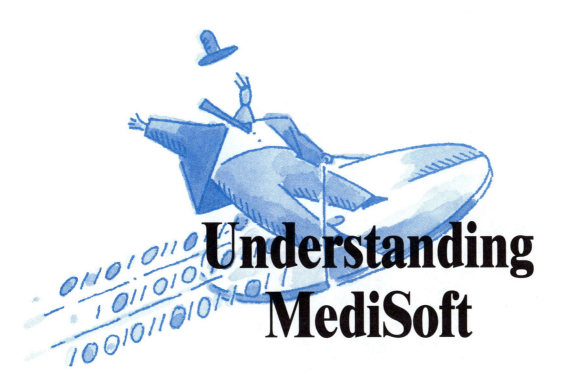

Understanding
MediSoft

SECTION 1

UNDERSTANDING THE MEDICAL OFFICE AND COMPUTERS

1 Introduction

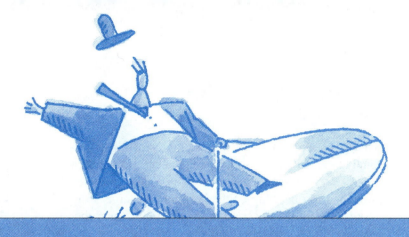

After completion of this chapter
you will be able to:

- Estimate the patient's portion of a bill.
- Complete a petty cash count slip.
- Set up a patient chart.

Let's begin! Today is January 14, CCYY, and you have just begun working for Consolidated Health Services (CHS), a large medical care facility. You, as a medical biller, keep patient accounts for a number of doctors. Patients of the offices are often seen by the same doctor each time (their primary care physician [PCP]), but if that PCP is unavailable, or if the patient needs a specialist, they may be referred to another provider within the office group.

After seeing the doctor, patients will often stop by the billing office on their way out to make a payment. At such times, the patient's claim information will be given to you, along with a Patient Information Sheet if necessary.

Sue Pervisor is the office manager, and your direct supervisor. Although you work in the same office as three other billers, they work on separate accounts. You are responsible for your own accounts.

Consolidated Health Services

CHS also owns an inpatient hospital facility. The hospital has an outpatient surgery wing, a lab and x-ray facility, and a separate urgent care trauma center. Attached to one wing of the hospital is a large drugstore that sells prescription medications, over-the-counter drugs, and some durable medical equipment.

CHS Ambulance Services is a sister company to Consolidated Health Services. Although it is a separate entity, it is owned by many of the same partners who own CHS. Because of this, the billing office also handles bills for the ambulance service.

As a medical biller for CHS, you are responsible for the billing of all doctors in the clinic, the ambulance company, and occasionally for bills from the hospital or drugstore (medical equipment charges). It is your responsibility to handle all billing for services rendered and to maintain patient accounts. You will bill the appropriate patients, insurance carriers, Medicare, or other entities responsible for payment; keep track of all patient accounts; make collection calls; and make bank deposits. You may also be asked to watch the front desk for a doctor's receptionist while she is at lunch or on break.

CHS has just begun using the MediSoft Patient Accounting system. Therefore, the system is new to you and all the other medical billers as well. It is your responsibility to set up the system and to learn how it works.

Collecting Payments from Patients

Most providers affiliated with CHS choose to collect the patient's portion of the bill after the insurance carrier has made payment. This allows the billing office to ask for payment from the patient one time only. However, Dr. Ben Dover requests that you estimate the patient's portion of the bill and collect this amount from the patient at the time services are rendered. To do this, you will need to estimate how much the insurance carrier will pay.

 Drew Blood, M.D., (General Practitioner)

 Reah E. Bright, M.D., (Radiologist)

 Noah Pulse, M.D., (Emergency Room)

 Kent Cure, M.D., (Emergency Room)

 Reed MiMind, M.D., (Psychiatrist)

 Phil Goode, M.D. (General Practitioner)

 Ben Dover, M.D., (Gastroenterologist)

 I.D. Liver, M.D., (Obstetrics/Gynecology)

 Allotta Payne, M.D., (Obstetrics/Gynecology)

 Anne S. Thesia, M.D., (Anesthesiologist)

 Yu B. Sickman, M.D., (General Practitioner)

 Butch M.N. Hackim, M.D., (Surgeon)

 Manny Kutz, M.D., (Assistant Surgeon)

 Will Kutteroff, M.D., (Surgeon)

First, contact the insurance carrier and determine the deductible amount for the patient, the percent covered by the insurance carrier, and any special payment circumstances. All this information should be placed on an Insurance Coverage Sheet (see Patient File Forms in Section 6).

The biller should contact the insurance carrier for subsequent visits to determine how much deductible has been previously paid by the patient and how much deductible is left to be paid. Because it is the beginning of the year, many patients will not have met their deductible. To estimate the patient's portion:

1. Subtract the amount of deductible previously met from the yearly deductible amount. This is the amount of deductible remaining to be paid.

2. Subtract the result of step 1 from the total amount of the charges for the visit. This amount will be covered by the insurance at a specified rate (i.e., 80%).

3. Multiply the result of step 2 by the patient's coinsurance amount. For example, if the insurance carrier pays 80%, then the patient's coinsurance is 20%.

4. Add the result of step 3 (patient's coinsurance) to the result of step 1 (unpaid deductible). This is the estimated patient responsibility for this bill.

Example: Johnny went to see the doctor for an ear infection. The total charges for services rendered

First Floor of Hospital

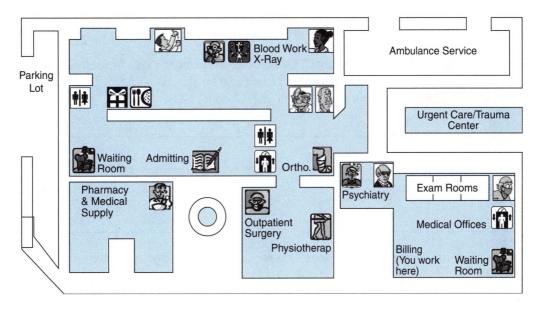

Second Floor of Hospital

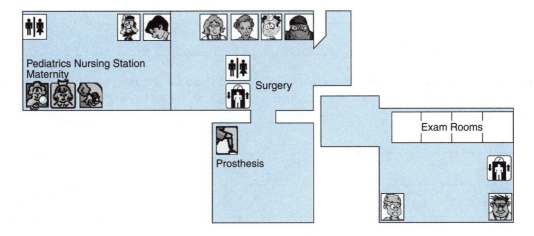

The third and fourth floors contain patient rooms and nursing stations

came to $145. You called the insurance carrier and were informed that Johnny's yearly deductible is $100. So far he has met $50.50 of his deductible. The insurance carrier pays 80%, and the patient's coinsurance is 20%.

1. $100 (deductible) − $50.50 (deductible paid) = $49.50 (unsatisfied deductible amount).

2. $145 (total charges) − $49.50 (unsatisfied deductible amount) = $95.50 (amount covered by insurance).

3. $95.50 (amount covered by insurance) × 20% (.20; patient coinsurance percentage) = $19.10 (patient's coinsurance amount).

4. $19.10 (patient's coinsurance amount) + $49.50 (unsatisfied deductible amount) = $68.60 (total patient responsibility).

Patients should be informed that additional payments might be necessary if the insurance carrier does not cover the full amount of the bill.

Exercise 1-1

Calculate the estimated patient portion for each of the following scenarios.

1. Abbie visited the doctor for measles treatment. The total charges came to $230. You called her insurance carrier, and they informed you that Abbie's deductible is $100. So far she has paid $23.25 of her deductible. The insurance carrier pays 80%, and the patient's coinsurance amount is 20%.

    1. _____

    2. _____

    3. _____

    4. _____

2. Bonnie went to the doctor for the mumps. The total charges came to $195. You called the insurance carrier and were informed that Bonnie's deductible is $150. So far she has met $15 of her deductible. The insurance carrier pays 90%.

    1. _____

    2. _____

    3. _____

    4. _____

3. Charlie went to the doctor for treatment for whooping cough. The total charges came to $115. You called the insurance carrier and were informed that his deductible is $125. So far he has met $5 of his deductible. The insurance carrier pays 80%.

    1. _____

    2. _____

    3. _____

    4. _____

4. Dick went to the doctor for chest pains. The total charges came to $263. You called the insurance carrier and were informed that Dick's deductible is $100. So far he has met $100. The insurance carrier pays 70%.

    1. _____

    2. _____

    3. _____

    4. _____

Some computerized billing systems will automatically multiply the amount of the visit by the patient's coinsurance portion. However, they will seldom calculate the amount of the deductible. Many offices prefer not to collect the deductible portion at the time services are rendered because it is possible that another claim for the patient will be processed by the insurance carrier prior to receipt of this claim. The deductible amount previously collected would then need to be refunded to the patient.

HIPAA

In 1996, President Clinton signed into law the Health Insurance Portability and Accountability Act (HIPAA). Here we will discuss the patient privacy and fraud and abuse issues.

The Act encompasses two main issues:

1. *Portability*; or the ability to transfer insurance companies and still be covered for preexisting conditions
2. *Accountability*; generally dealing with the patient's right to privacy from the medical provider, health insurer, and any other parties required in the healthcare process (i.e., billers, clearinghouses, and so on)

Regarding the privacy section of HIPAA, the Department of Health and Human Services states

> *The privacy requirements limit the release of patient Protected Health Information (PHI) without the patient's knowledge and consent beyond that required for patient care. Patient's personal information must be more securely guarded and more carefully handled when conducting the business of health care.*

All healthcare entities were required to meet the standards set in the privacy issues section of HIPAA by April 14, 2003.

The following are the general rules for ensuring that privacy guidelines are met:

1. Always obtain an authorization to release information before releasing any information. Most releases routinely signed in the medical practice only authorize the physician to release information necessary to process a patient's claim. Additional authorization should be obtained to release any information to other parties. These releases should state exactly what information is to be released, the dates of any services provided that fall within the release, the person to whom the information may be released, the signature of the patient, the date of the signature, and the date the release expires.
2. Make sure that a release was signed by the member prior to processing a claim. If possible, ask the provider for a copy of the patient's signature on the release form. This will ensure that you have the right to look at the information contained on the claim.
3. Gather only the information that is necessary and relevant to the billing or processing of the claim.
4. Use only legal and ethical means to collect the information required. Whenever permission is necessary, obtain written authorization from the insured or claimant (guardian or parent if the claimant is a minor).
5. When requested, and subject to any applicable legal or ethical prohibition or privilege, the insured or claimant concerned should be advised of the nature and general uses to be made of the information.
6. Make every reasonable effort to ensure that the information on which an action is based is accurate, relevant, timely, and complete.
7. On request, the claimant or insured should be given the opportunity to correct or clarify the information given by or about him or her, and the file should be amended to the extent that it is fair to both the insurer and the member or claimant. Requests for review or clarification of medical information will be accepted only from the healthcare provider from whom the information was obtained.
8. In general, disclosures of information to a third party (other than those described to the insured or claimant) should be made only with the written authorization of the member or claimant. This includes disclosure to employers, family members, or former spouses.
9. All practical precautions should be taken to ensure that claim files are physically secure and that access to the use of such files is limited to authorized personnel. This includes not leaving files out, locking all files, and even turning your computer screen away from where it might be seen by other persons. Security passwords and other security measures may also be required, depending on your office situation.
10. All personnel involved in the processing of claims should be advised of the need to protect the right of privacy in obtaining required information and the need to treat all individually identifiable information as confidential. Willful abuse of the privacy of any insured or claimant by the employee may be cause for dismissal.
11. The disclosure of a diagnosis should never be made to a member or his or her family. If the member requests this information, refer the member to the physician. There may be a reason the patient does not know his or her diagnosis.

12. Never release any information to an ex-spouse. This includes the member's address, phone number, when a claim was paid, to whom, and other information. The ex-spouse should be instructed to contact the member directly.

13. Do not leave files, members' records, or appointment books open on your desk or in an area where they may be seen by others. This includes member files or information that may be displayed on a computer screen. The best way to handle this is to be sure that all files are closed or are turned over on your desk. Computer screens must be placed in a position so that they cannot be seen by anyone passing by. If necessary, use a screen saver or other unrestricted document that can be clicked on to replace the one you are working on instantaneously.

14. If a minor patient has the legal right to authorize treatment for services, then disclosure to the parents, legal guardians of the minor, or other persons may be a violation of HIPAA or the confidentiality of Medical Information Privacy and Security Act (MIPSA).

15. Be cautious about releasing information to a patient's employer, even if an authorization to release information has been obtained.

If in doubt as to whether specific information should be released, check with your supervisor before, not after, releasing it.

These guidelines cover some of the basic aspects of HIPAA privacy regulations. For detailed information regarding HIPAA guidelines, complete rules and regulations regarding HIPAA can be found online at www.hipaa.org.

Setting Up Your "Office"

Each person going through this text will be responsible for setting up their own office and completing each of the exercises. For this reason it is important to maintain a set of files and other work items that can be used day to day. Setting up your "office" with the following items will help to keep them neat and ensure that items are easily accessible.

You will need the following items to properly complete the exercises in this book:

- 2 Envelopes (one for petty cash/payments and one for deposits made).

- 15 family/patient file folders (see Patient Files section later).
- 1 "practice" folder for keeping all daily charts and forms that are generated for the practice.
- 1 folder for all completed claims that would be sent to the insurance carrier.
- 110 1500 Health Insurance Claim forms for billing.
- 5 UB-92 forms for billing.
- 1 expanding file folder for keeping all of the preceding items together.
- Pens and pencils.

Additionally you will need access to the following:

- Current Procedural Terminology (CPT®), International Classification of Diseases, Ninth Edition (ICD-9-CM), and Healthcare Common Procedure Coding System (HCPCS) coding books
- Scissors
- 2-hole punch
- Medical dictionary and/or other reference books

Place the cash and deposit envelopes in the front of the expanding folder, followed by the practice folder and then the patient charts. As you are introduced to each patient and/or their family, create a family chart and place it in your expanding file folder. All other forms for setting up your office are located in **Patient File Forms—Section 6**.

Petty Cash and Deposit Envelope

As a medical biller, you are responsible for keeping a petty cash envelope and for reconciling the amount in petty cash and the amount collected from patients. At the end of each day you will prepare a deposit slip with all payments received during that day. You should recount the petty cash to ensure that the same amount remains at the end of the day as there was at the beginning; also be sure that the money in petty cash is sufficient for making change for customers.

It is suggested that you keep all petty cash and payments received in a single envelope. When a patient makes a payment, place the check or cash into the envelope. If change is needed, remove the proper change from the envelope. A second envelope should be used for deposits. Clearly label the envelopes **CASH ENVELOPE** and **DEPOSITS MADE**.

Section 5 contains simulated petty cash for the cash drawer and forms used for petty cash. Cut out each of the bills and coins and place them in your Cash Envelope. Using a copy of the Petty Cash Count slip, determine the amount of money in your petty cash drawer. Your count should always include the paper currency, all coins, and petty cash receipts. This slip should be used each time you reconcile petty cash. During the Simulated Work Program—Section 3, use a.m. to designate the first counting of petty cash at the beginning of the day and p.m. to designate the count at the end of the day.

1. How much money is in your petty cash envelope?

_____

Additionally, supervisors such as Sue Pervisor may take up to $20 from petty cash to cover small items needed for the office. Each should sign a petty cash receipt (see **Patient File Forms—Section 6**) showing the date the money was taken, the amount, and what the money was used for. After purchases are made, the receipt and any change left over should be returned to the petty cash drawer. Be sure that the amount of the receipt and the change total the amount that was originally given.

Patient Files

The patient files are also kept in your office. CHS keeps family files for their patients, instead of individual files. Each family file consists of a three- or four-page file folder with pronged paper fasteners at the top for holding information (**see Figure 1–1**). Each file should contain information in the following order:

Fastener 1

1. Patient Information Sheet. (The bottom section of the patient information sheet includes an Authorization to Release Information and an Assignment of Benefits.)

2. Insurance Coverage Sheet. (This form will be completed and inserted during the Simulated Work Program).

3. Any other forms or information that pertains to the entire family.

Fastener 2

1. Billing information (1500 Health Insurance claims and patient statements) in reverse chronological order (most recent date first) for the insured. These will be completed during the exercises and simulated work program in this text.

Fasteners 3, 4, and 5

1. Billing information, 1500 Health Insurance claims, and patient statements in chronological order (most recent first) for dependents. Each dependent should have their own separate fastener.

2. If there are more than three dependents in the family, insert a divider or folder with fasteners to accommodate the additional family members.

Last Fastener

1. For training purposes, this page will be used to attach all items that are given to the patient or insured. These items can include change for a cash payment, a receipt, or statements that were sent to the patient.

Patient files should be kept available at all times.

Training Tip

For class purposes, you may want to create patient files by placing one manila folder inside another and securing them together at the fold. Then attach a two-pronged paper fastener at the top of each page to hold the papers in place. Keep all your files in an expanding file folder.

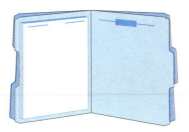

■ **Figure 1–1**

CHAPTER REVIEW

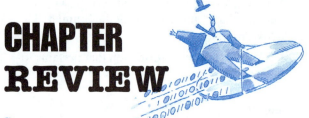

- With practice you will become proficient at these skills and acquire many more, making you a valuable member of CHS.

Summary

- As a medical biller at Consolidated Health Services you have numerous responsibilities. Some of those responsibilities include setting up and maintaining patient billing information, estimating the patient portion of charges, and reconciling petty cash.

Questions for Review

Directions: Answer the following questions without looking back into the material just covered. Write your answers in the space provided.

1. What is the purpose of a petty cash receipt?

   _____

   _____

2. Name two uses for petty cash.

   1. _____

      _____

   2. _____

      _____

3. What does HIPAA stand for, and what is its purpose?

   _____

   _____

   _____

4. List the four steps for estimating the patient's portion of a bill.

1. _____

_____

2. _____

_____

3. _____

_____

4. _____

_____

5. What items are placed on side three of the family chart?

_____

_____

If you were unable to answer any of the questions, refer back to that section, and then fill in the answers.

2

Computers—A Quick Review

After completion of this chapter
you will be able to:

- List the three main components of a computer
- Describe the keyboard and demonstrate its use.
- Define commonly used computer terms.

In today's world, computers are a common part of life. They are used in nearly every business and in many home environments. In the medical community, computers are used extensively for billing patients, handling patient accounting, and handling the provider's accounts and correspondence.

Computer Terminology

With the development of computers, a whole new set of terms had to be created to define items relating to the application and use of these machines. Although "computerese" is a complete language that could take years to understand, most people who use computers will only need to be familiar with some of the terms. The most common of terms include the following.

Backup—A backup copy is a duplicate file or set of information contained in a different area of the computer or on magnetic tape or disk. This allows you to recreate information if something should happen to your main file.

Batch—A group of documents, papers, or forms that are related in some way, often by date or batch number. Unrelated papers or claims may be put together in a batch and given a specific number.

Bit—Binary digit, the smallest possible unit of memory storage. Eight bits is equal to one byte.

Bug—A computer program error. Bugs can cause a program to work improperly or not at all.

Byte—A measurement for the storage capacity of computers. A byte is equal to eight bits, or roughly the amount of bits needed to make one character or letter.

Central Processing Unit (CPU)—The brains of a computer. It controls the internal memory and directs the processing and flow of information.

Command Key—A key or combination of keys that activates a command in a computer program.

Cursor—A small light, bar, or flashing line on the computer screen that indicates the position of the next data entry.

Database—A collection of electronically stored data organized so that its contents can easily be accessed, managed and updated.

Debug—To remove errors from a computer or a software program.

Disk—A device for storing information. There are two main types of disks: hard and floppy.

Disk, Hard—A disk made of hard material that can be stored inside the computer housing or outside, attached securely by cables and wires.

Disk, Floppy—A plastic diskette that holds data information and is easily transportable. Floppy disks are often 3.5 inches square. However, compact discs (CDs) and various flash memory storage devices are replacing 3.5 inch disks, as they are easier to transport, are more durable, and can hold more information.

Documentation—An instruction book detailing how to use a computer program.

DOS—Disk Operating System. A set of programmed instructions, which commands the computer's operation.

Downtime—The time during which a computer is not operating properly.

Footer—A notation that appears at the bottom of a page or computer screen.

Format—The way the data is organized or how it appears. Format can include whether items are presented in upper- or lowercase; numbered or lettered; left, center, or right aligned; width of margins; and many other factors.

Hard Copy—A printout of information from the computer.

Hardware—The pieces or components of a computer system. These can include the monitor, keyboard, hard disk, computer housing, or modem.

Header—A notation that appears at the top of a page or computer screen.

Input—To enter information into a computer.

Input Device—Items such as the keyboard or mouse that are used to interact with the computer.

Interface—The linking of two or more computer systems (i.e., computer to computer, or computer to printer).

K (kilobyte)—A unit of memory storage measurement. A kilobyte is equal to 1,000 bytes. For example, a computer may have 640 K of memory.

Memory—The computer's ability to store data.

Menu—A list of items or computer functions displayed on a computer screen from which the operator can choose.

Modem—A device that converts outgoing digital data into sound waves so it can be transmitted across telephone lines and that can reconvert incoming sound waves into digital data. Most computers have a built-in "internal" modem.

Mouse—A handheld device used to control the video display of a computer.

Network—An interconnection of computers.

On-line System—(1) A system in which data is input directly into the computer, and output data is sent directly from the computer to where it is used (i.e., printer, modem). (2) A system that works without human intervention between the recording and the processing of material.

Optical Character Recognition (OCR)—A device that can read typed characters and convert them to computer data.

Program—Another word for software; a set of instructions that can be loaded into the computer. It commands the computer on how to work to achieve the purposes of the program (i.e., Medi-Soft is a program for medical patient accounting and billing).

Prompt—A symbol (often >) that indicates the computer is ready to receive information.

RAM (Random Access Memory)—A data storage system in which data may be stored randomly, and retrieved by specifying its location.

Retrieve—The act of locating a stored file and bringing it up on screen.

ROM (Read-Only Memory)—A data storage system in which information can be read, but not changed. This usually includes permanent programs.

Scrolling—The ability to move from one side of the screen to another, top to bottom, or page by page through a document.

Soft Copy—The information displayed on a computer screen. The printing of this data onto paper is called a hard copy.

Software—Another word for computer program.

Sort—The process by which a computer arranges data in a specified order.

Spooling—A device whereby the output from a computer is placed in storage queues to await transmission to a device that moves slower than the computer output (i.e., the storage of data to a file until it can be read by a printer with a more limited memory capacity).

Terminal—A device or system that can receive information from and send information to a computer system.

Time-Sharing—The use of a computer device for more than one purpose at one time (i.e., working on one document while another is being sent to the printer) or the use of a system by more than one user at one time.

Voice Activation—The ability of a computer device to recognize and respond to verbal commands.

The Computer

There are three main components to a computer, the central processing unit, the monitor, and the input/output (I/O) devices. The central processing unit is enclosed in a box that houses the memory and functional components of the computer. The monitor is the screen connected to the computer that allows you to see the program and the data you are working with. Input/output devices are used to interface and communicate with the computer. The most common input/output device is the keyboard. The input commands and data are typed through the keyboard.

Because the keyboard is the main component used to enter data, we will describe it in more detail. There are five main parts of a keyboard: the angle adjustment, the alpha keypad, the numeric keypad, the shortcut keys, and the function keys.

The keyboard angle adjustment consists of two small legs that are located under the back of the keyboard. Pushing these up or down allows you to adjust the keyboard to two different positions.

The alpha keypad looks and works like a standard typewriter keyboard. There are alphabetic, numeric, and symbol keys, as well as those for spacing and capitalizing letters.

The numeric keypad is usually located on the right-hand side of the keyboard and performs a dual function. With the Num Lock key engaged, it is used for the rapid entry of numbers. Without engaging Num Lock, the keypad can be used the same as the shortcut keys.

Between the alpha keypad and the numeric keypad are the shortcut keys. These keys allow you to move more quickly through a document. These can include the following keys:

- **Home:** Moves you to the beginning of the line the cursor is on.
- **End:** Moves you to the end of the line the cursor is on.
- **Page Up:** Moves you up one page in the current document.
- **Page Down:** Moves you down one page in the current document.
- **Delete:** Deletes characters typed to the right of where the cursor is.
- **Insert:** New characters typed in will replace the existing characters shown on the screen.
- **Arrow Keys:** These keys allow you to move the cursor one space to the right, left, up, or down in the document.

Function keys allow complex program commands to be performed with a single keystroke. The 12 function keys are located along the top or on the left side of the keyboard. Different software programs use the function keys for different purposes. To properly use them, consult the user manual for the specific program you are working with.

Using the Computer

Different computer systems use different keys to produce the same results. Often if you have mastered one computer system, you will find a related computer system to be fairly easy to learn.

Choosing **main menu options** is the same as choosing a main heading on a restaurant menu. Do you want a main dish today or a salad? Do you want to edit information, or print reports? To choose a main menu option, click on the menu choice at the top of the screen.

Once you have chosen a main menu option, a **submenu option** menu will appear on the screen. Submenu options give you different choices that have been grouped under the main heading. For example, if you chose a salad from the main menu, which type of salad do you prefer, Chinese chicken or chef's salad? If you have chosen to print reports, do you want to print an insurance aging report or a patient ledger?

Disk drives are where the data on your computer is stored. Most personal computers have a **hard drive** installed within the computer. This is most commonly called the C drive. The A and D drives are located on the front of the computer (though some computers only have an A drive installed). The A and D disk drives have a slot through which you can slide a **floppy disk** or **CD**.

A floppy disk is a circular piece of magnetic film that is enclosed in a square plastic holder. When you store information to your disk (i.e., to the A or B drive), you are actually instructing the computer to record the information in your document onto the magnetic film. This is very similar to recording a voice on a cassette tape.

The magnetic field contained in these disks is very sensitive and should be handled carefully. The following rules should be observed when dealing with data diskettes:

1. Never touch the magnetic media housed inside the plastic cover or on the back of the CD.

2. Store all disks or CDs inside a plastic or paper cover to protect them. Insert and remove the disk or CD carefully from the cover to prevent scratching the magnetic media.

3. Keep diskettes stored at temperatures between 50 degrees and 125 degrees Fahrenheit. Never leave a data disk exposed to sunlight.

4. Keep all magnets away from your data disks. Information is stored on a magnetic media, which can be erased when it comes in contact with a magnet. This includes the magnet contained in office supplies such as paper clip holders.

5. Before touching a data disk, discharge any static electricity you may have picked up by touching a piece of metal or an antistatic mat. Static electricity will also demagnetize items and therefore erase the data contained on a disk.

6. To prevent any changes to stored information, cover the "write protect" notch on the side of the disk. On a 3.5-inch disk, this notch can be closed by sliding a small plastic square to cover the hole.

7. Do not write on a disk label with a ballpoint pen or pencil; rather, use a felt-tip marker. The pressure applied when writing with pen or pencil may cause impressions on the magnetic media damaging the content.

When information is stored on a disk, the disk can be taken from one computer to another and the data used wherever you would like.

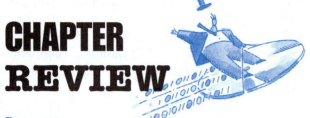

CHAPTER REVIEW

Summary

- Computers have infiltrated all aspects of business life, including the medical office. Using the computer saves time, produces neater and cleaner reports, reduces errors, and allows for electronic submission of data to the insurance carrier.

- Learning to use a computer program quickly and accurately and learning the proper means of storing information is important to become a proficient medical biller.

Questions for Review

Directions: Answer the following questions without looking back into the material just covered. Write your answers in the space provided.

1. List the three main components of a computer system and define their use.

    1. _____

    2. _____

    3. _____

2. List the five main parts of the keyboard and define their use.

    1. _____

    2. _____

    3. _____

    4. _____

    5. _____

3. What does it mean to "back up" your data?

_____

_____

4. The cursor is

_____

_____

5. Define the following terms:

RAM

_____

ROM

_____

Menu

_____

Mouse

_____

If you are unable to answer any of these questions, refer back to that section in the chapter, and then fill in the answers.

3
Using MediSoft

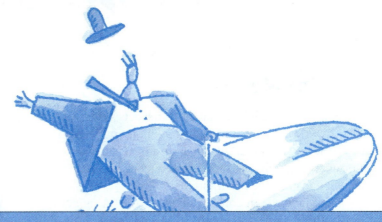

After completion of this chapter
you will be able to:

- Enter and exit the MediSoft program.
- Access submenu options under the menu bar.
- Access menu bar options and select a menu option.
- Operate the function keys.

MediSoft is one of the most comprehensive and popular computerized medical billing software programs available today. The MediSoft Patient Accounting System not only creates claims for billing insurance carriers, but also keeps track of patient accounts and creates many of the forms necessary for the efficient running of a medical office.

Due to the constant revision of MediSoft, you may not have the most recent version. In this text we have given you information for the latest version of MediSoft, but we have also included descriptions of menus, fields, and options that are found in earlier versions. The differences among versions are often small and involve renaming a field or repositioning a field within a screen. As you go through your software with this text, keep in mind that something that has been renamed in the new version will most likely have the same function as in the old version.

This text is based on the concept that you learn by doing. Therefore, as you read about each function and field in the MediSoft system, you will also be asked to enter data into these fields. It is important that you take your time and enter the data correctly, as it will be used in the simulated work program. If data has been incorrectly entered here, it may adversely affect reports, charges, or other entries that are completed during the simulated work program.

It takes practice to use a computer program quickly and effectively. Do not rush through the exercises. Although you will have the opportunity to enter data in each of the screens, these exercises are meant to familiarize you with the screens. Do not worry if you do not feel totally comfortable with the screen. You will gain additional practice using each of the screens during the simulated work program.

Entering MediSoft

To begin using MediSoft, you must first access the system. You should have a MediSoft icon on your screen with the word *MediSoft* underneath. Using your mouse, double-click on the MediSoft icon. The system will then display the MediSoft main screen.

The main screen consists of Menu Bars arranged across the top of the screen. A second level shows icons for accessing specific tools in the MediSoft program.

Menu Bar

Let's become familiar with the Menu Bar (**see Figure 3–1**) and its options. MediSoft contains both a Menu Bar, to bring up a menu of options, and a Tool Bar, for quick access to some of the MediSoft operations. There are nine menu operations as follows:

1. File
2. Edit
3. Activities
4. Lists
5. Reports
6. Tools
7. Window
8. Services
9. Help

When you want to access an item in the Menu Bar, you have two options:

1. Use your mouse to move the arrow to the menu choice and click the button once; or
2. Hold down the Alt key and press the letter that is underlined for each of the menu options.

Accessing each of the choices in the Menu Bar allows you to see the submenu items that can be chosen in that menu option. A list of choices will pop up on the screen from which you may choose. To enter a menu choice, access the option by using either of the two methods mentioned earlier.

Start your computer and enter the MediSoft program. Click on each of the following menu choices as they are discussed, and answer the questions asked. Remember that different versions will vary. Some

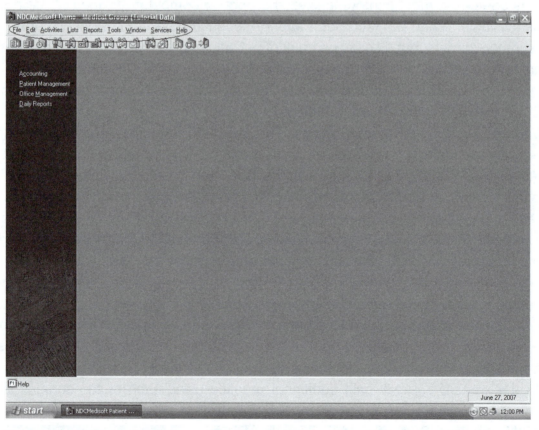

■ **Figure 3–1** Menu Bar

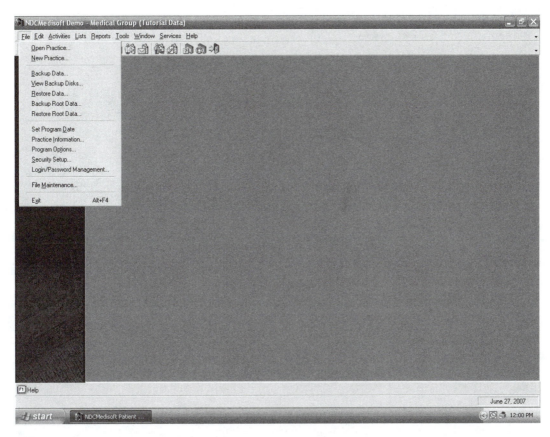

■ Figure 3–2   File Menu

menus may have fewer choices than there are lines to be filled, depending on your version of MediSoft.

The **File Menu (see Figure 3–2)** allows the user to enter data regarding the office, back up and restore data, program options, and maintain files. The File Menu's submenu choices are

1. Open Practice
2. New Practice
3. Backup Data
4. View Backup Disks
5. Restore Data
6. Backup Root Data
7. Restore Root Data
8. Set Program Date
9. Practice Information
10. Program Options
11. Security Setup
12. Login/Password Management
13. File Maintenance
14. Exit

The **Edit Menu (see Figure 3–3)** is for editing items. These are usually text items. List the submenu choices for the Edit Menu in the following spaces.

1. _____

2. _____

3. _____

4. _____

The **Activities Menu (see Figure 3–4)** provides an opportunity to enter transactions (billings and payment receipts) and appointments. These are the screens that will be used most often in daily practice.

List the submenu choices in the Activities Menu in the following spaces.

1. _____

2. _____

3. _____

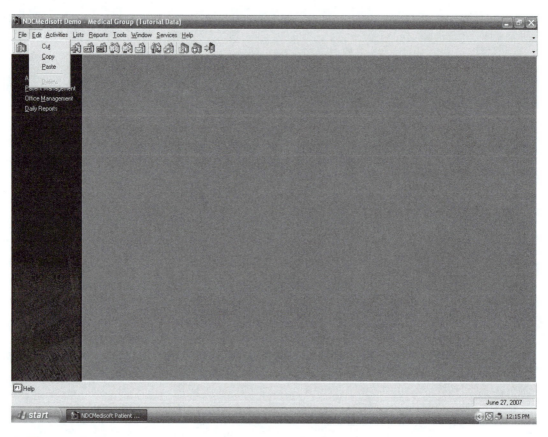

■ Figure 3–3 Edit Menu

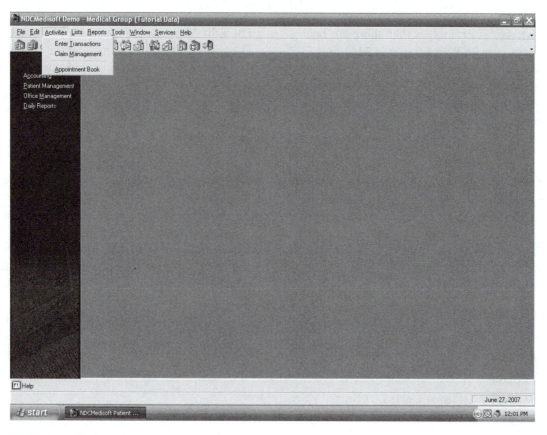

■ Figure 3–4 Activities Menu

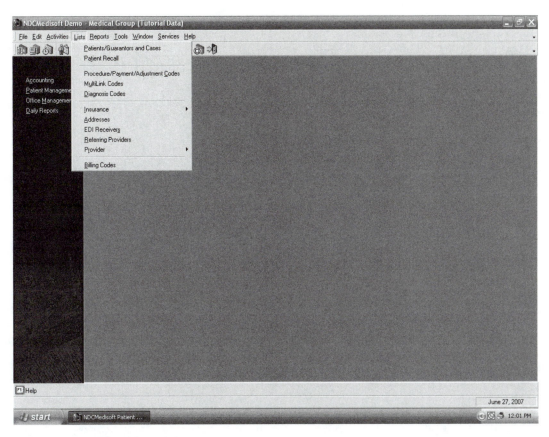

■ Figure 3–5   Lists Menu

The **Lists Menu (see Figure 3–5)** gives you access to lists of those people and entities your practice does business with. These lists usually include names, addresses, and phone numbers, as well as other pertinent data. List the submenu choices in the Lists Menu in the following spaces.

1. _____

2. _____

3. _____

4. _____

5. _____

6. _____

   A. _____

7. _____

8. _____

9. _____

10. _____

   A. _____

   B. _____

11. _____

The **Reports Menu (see Figure 3–6)** allows you to print reports on both the patient and the office. These reports help you keep track of how the practice is doing. List in the following spaces the submenu choices in the Reports Menu, including the options given through side arrows.

1. _____

   A. _____

   B. _____

   C. _____

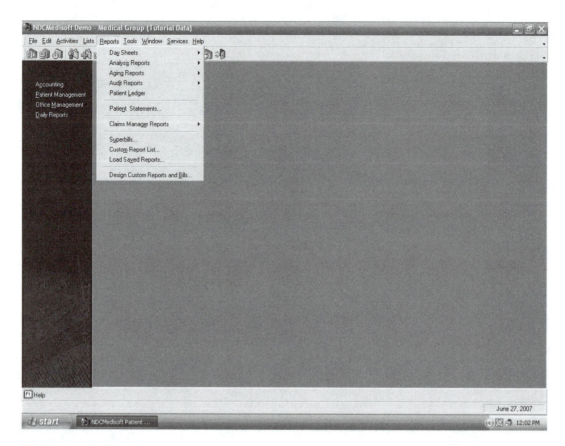

■ Figure 3–6 Reports Menu

2. _____

   A. _____

3. _____

   A. _____

   B. _____

   C. _____

   D. _____

   E. _____

4. _____

   A. _____

   B. _____

5. _____

6. _____

7. _____

   A. _____

   B. _____

8. _____

9. _____

10. _____

11. _____

The **Tools Menu (see Figure 3–7***)* gives you access to additional tools that might be helpful in making the practice run smoothly.

   List the submenu choices for the Tools Menu in the following spaces.

1. _____

2. _____

3. _____

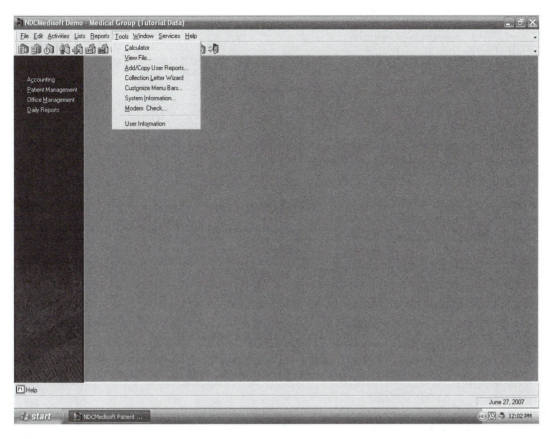

■ **Figure 3–7**   Tools Menu

4. _____

5. _____

6. _____

7. _____

8. _____

The **Window Menu (see Figure 3–8)** allows you to close, minimize, or sort all open windows. List the submenu choices in the Window Menu in the following spaces.

1. _____

2. _____

3. _____

4. _____

5. _____

The **Services Menu (see Figure 3–9)** offers a link to an online resource that allows a practice to write prescriptions over the Internet. These prescriptions can be transmitted to nearby pharmacies, allowing patients to pick up their prescriptions quickly.

List the submenu choices in the Services Menu.

1. _____

2. _____

The **Help Menu (see Figure 3–10)** allows you to access additional information on using MediSoft. List the submenu choices in the Help Menu in the following spaces, including the options given through side arrows.

1. _____

2. _____

3. _____

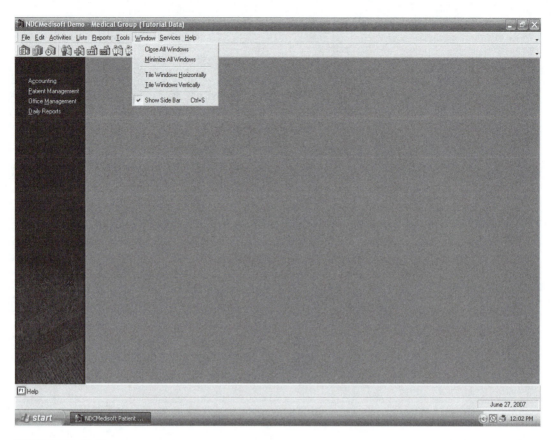

■ **Figure 3–8** Window Menu

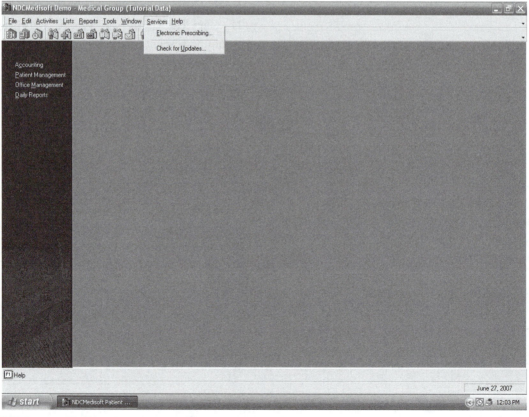

■ **Figure 3–9** Services Menu

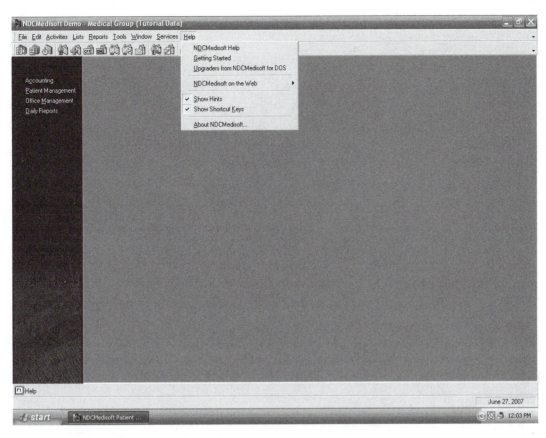

■ **Figure 3–10**   Help Menu

4. _____

   A. _____

   B. _____

   C. _____

   D. _____

   E. _____

5. _____

6. _____

7. _____

Tool Bar

The Tool Bar (**see Figure 3–11**) is used to quickly access functions. For example, the first icon in the tool bar is for Transaction Entry. To enter transactions click on this icon, or you can click on the Activities Menu, and then choose Enter Transactions.

As you move the mouse arrow to each of the icons, their function will be highlighted both at the site of the icon and at the bottom of the screen.

For example, the second icon is Claim Management. The wording near the icon says Claim Management. The description at the bottom of the page says, "Use this window to print and send insurance claims."

Use your mouse to move the arrow to each of the icons on the Tool Bar. Allow the mouse arrow to rest on the icon a moment. List the wording that appears near the icon and at the bottom of the screen in the following chart. (If no wording appears near your icon, this option may be turned off. To turn it on, click on the Help Menu, and then choose the Show Hints submenu option. This is an on/off key. A check mark by the option means the hints will be shown. No check means the hints will not show.)

ICON   **Identify the ICON and the message that appears at the bottom of the screen.**

_____

_____

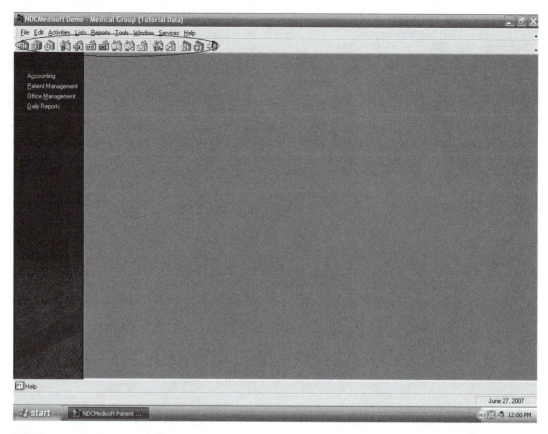

■ **Figure 3–11** Tool Bar

_____

_____

_____

Sidebar Options

If the option to show Sidebar **(see Figure 3–12)** has been checked, your screen may show four subject tabs vertically arranged on the left side of the screen. These are

1. Accounting
2. Patient Management
3. Office Management
4. Daily Reports

Clicking on these tabs opens a menu of more specific options under each heading. These submenu options are the same as those accessed through the main menu bar. Click on each option and list the submenu options in the following spaces.

The **Accounting sidebar (see Figure 3–13)** allows you to perform accounting functions. List the submenu options found on the Accounting sidebar.

1. _____

2. _____

The **Patient Management sidebar (see Figure 3–14)** allows you to access options that deal with managing the practice's patients. List the submenu options found on the Patient Management sidebar.

1. _____

2. _____

3. _____

4. _____

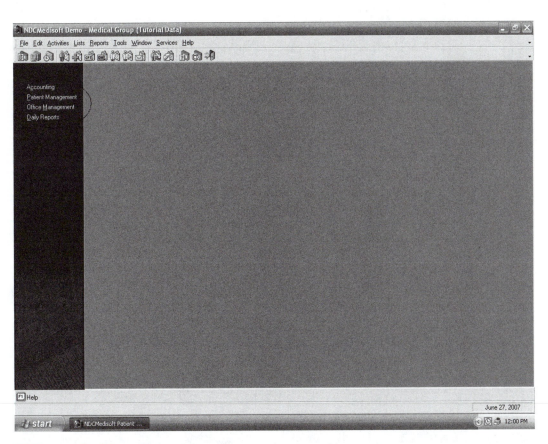

■ Figure 3–12 Sidebar Options

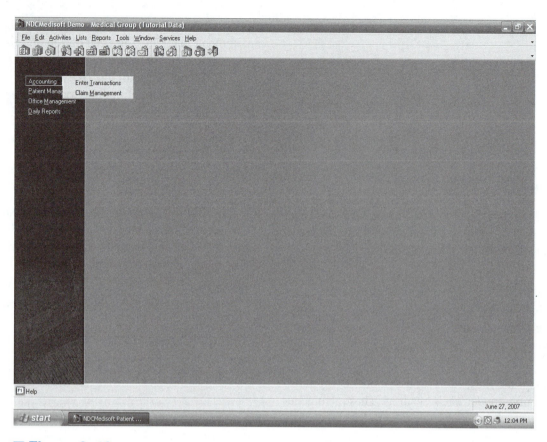

■ **Figure 3–13**   Accounting Sidebar

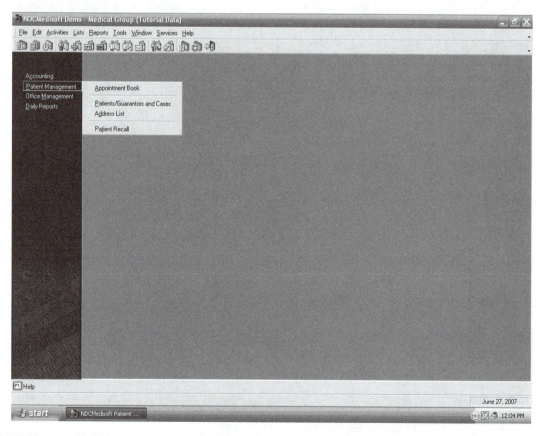

■ **Figure 3–14**   Patient Management Sidebar

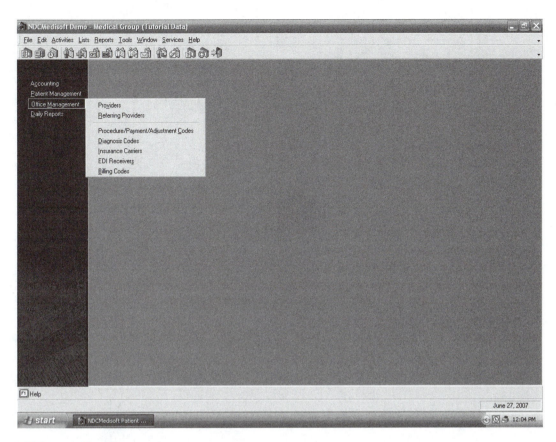

■ **Figure 3–15**   Office Management Sidebar

The **Office Management sidebar (see Figure 3–15)** allows you to access functions that help the office to run smoothly. List the submenu options in the Office Management sidebar.

1. _____

2. _____

3. _____

4. _____

5. _____

6. _____

7. _____

The **Daily Reports sidebar (see Figure 3–16)** allows you to print reports that are used on a daily basis. List the submenu options in the Daily Reports sidebar.

1. _____

2. _____

3. _____

General Functions and Keys

The following functions and keys work on many screens throughout the menus in the MediSoft Patient Accounting system. In MediSoft the available function keys are shown in the command line at the bottom of the screen. They can be used in virtually any screen.

F1—Help. Pressing this key will give you more information regarding the field that is currently highlighted by the cursor. You may also access this option by clicking on the Help tool bar icon or the Help Menu Option.

F3—Save. The information entered into each field is not saved until the **F3** key is pressed. This saves the information onto the hard drive and allows it to be retrieved at a later date. If you do not press **F3** at the end of a screen or click on the save button, your data will be lost when you leave that screen.

F6—Search. The search option is available to search name and description fields. It is not available for use in most numbered fields. The search function works for any string of letters that matches those that are entered. Therefore, if you enter the letters "Jack" in the

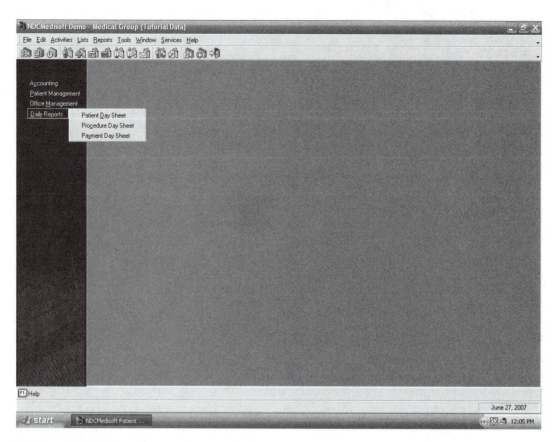

■ Figure 3–16   Daily Reports Sidebar

patient chart/name field, the computer will bring up everything with this string of letters in the beginning of the last name, including Thomas Jack-man and Bob Jackson. If you enter a single letter, the computer locates all records that contain that letter in the beginning of a word. Thus, entering "A" in the procedures screen will bring up adjustment, but not cash.

You may also access the search field by clicking on the magnifying glass, which is found to the right of many fields.

Pressing **F2** while in the search mode will allow you to search a different index option. For example, in the Procedure Code Information screen, pressing **F2** will search the code number rather than the description of the procedure. Once you have entered the search screen, the bottom of your screen will tell you whether the **F2** option is available for this screen and which field will be searched if you press the **F2** key.

F7—Ledger. Pressing F7 opens the Quick Ledger window. This window allows you to look at the account of the patient you are currently working on.

F8—New. This key allows you to enter new information into an appropriate screen. A few fields allow you to switch from one screen to another quickly to add necessary information. For example, if you are working on the Transaction Entry screen and attempt to enter a diagnosis that has not been previously entered into the Diagnosis Code database, pressing **F8** will allow you to quickly access the Diagnosis Code Entry screen. After entering the information on the diagnosis code, pressing **F3** (save) will take you back to the Transaction Entry screen. The information you have just entered into the Diagnosis Code Entry screen will appear in the diagnosis field on the Transaction Entry screen.

F9—Edit. This key will allow you to edit or change data that has already been saved.

F11—Quick Balance. This key will allow you to see balance information for the chosen guarantor. Often the guarantor is the insured. Using this window will allow you to see all balances for the insured and their dependents.

F12—Office Messenger. This key opens the NDC MediSoft Office Messenger program. This allows you to send a quick message to someone else using the program.

The **F1**, **F6**, and **F8** keys are context sensitive. This means that choosing them will only access files that are related to the current position of the cursor. Therefore, if your cursor is in the Diagnosis Code position, the Help key will tell you about that field only, the Search key will search only for diagnosis codes, etc.

Esc—Exits you from the screen or field you are in and takes you back to the previous menu. Be sure to save prior to pressing **Esc** if you wish to keep your data.

Enter—Enters the information into the current field you are working on and moves the cursor to the next entry field.

Space—Hitting the space bar will check or uncheck a box when your cursor is in the box.

Arrow Keys—The up and down arrow keys (↑ and ↓) will move the cursor up or down to the previous or the next field on the screen.

The left and right arrow keys (← and →) will move the cursor to the right and left within the field you are currently in.

End—The End key will move the cursor to the end of the field you are currently working in.

Home—The Home key will move you to the beginning of the field you are currently working in.

Tab—The Tab key will move the cursor around the screen. This is the key that should be used when you have finished entering data in one field and wish to move on to the next field. If you press Enter after completing a field, in many of the screens MediSoft will assume you have completed the entry and wish to exit that screen.

There are other function keys that only work in a specific menu. For example, the F2 key will open the MultiLink window if you are in the Transaction Entry screen. In the List Windows screen the same F2 key will change the value in the field.

Because the function of these keys is specific to a certain field, they will not be discussed here.

The MediSoft Icon

The MediSoft Icon in the upper-left-hand corner of the screen has additional menu options. Clicking on this icon will list a menu of these options. In previous versions, a—Box occupied the upper-left-hand corner of the screen. The function remains the same.

Minimize and maximize allow you to change the size of the screen you are looking at. Minimize will make it very small. Maximize will enlarge it to fill the entire screen.

Close will end this application and return you to the previous screen or a blank screen. This is the way to exit an application. Although hitting **F3** (save) will automatically exit you from some applications, it should not be used if you have not entered any data into the application. Otherwise you will be saving blank screens, thus using memory storage space.

CHAPTER REVIEW

Summary

- The MediSoft Patient Accounting system has a wide variety of menus and screens, which provide most functions needed for handling patient accounting. Learning the various operations menus and the items contained within those menus is essential to being able to run the MediSoft program efficiently and effectively.

- Some keys function the same throughout all MediSoft menus and fields. Learning these keys and how they function will greatly aid in improving data entry time and ease in operating the computer.

Questions for Review

Directions: Answer the following questions without looking back into the material just covered. Write your answers in the space provided.

1. In which menu sidebar option will you find the Enter Transactions submenu choice?

_____

_____

2. What is the name of the menu sidebar option to access the screen for entering patient data into the computer?

_____

_____

3. Which key is used to get more information or "help" on how to fill out a particular field?

_____

_____

4. Which key is used to save your data?

_____

_____

5. What are the three ways of initiating a search?

1. _____

_____

2. _____

_____

3. _____

_____

6. In which menu bar option will you find the Patient Ledger submenu choice?

_____

_____

7. In which menu bar option will you find the Insurance Carriers List submenu choice?

_____

_____

8. In which menu sidebar option will you find the Appointment Book submenu choice?

_____

_____

9. In which menu bar option will you find the Backup Data submenu choice?

_____

_____

10. What function does the **F8** key perform? _____

_____

_____

If you were unable to answer any of the questions, refer back to that section, and then fill in the answers.

4
File Menu Options

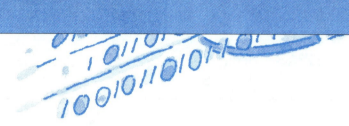

After completion of this chapter
you will be able to:

- Set up a practice, set program date, and enter new patient information.

- Restore data, purge unnecessary data, and rebuild your data files.

Now let's actually begin entering data into the system. We will go through each of the menu options one by one. In each you will be asked to enter or change data. Follow the directions exactly and complete each step before moving on to the next. If you skip items, your data could be adversely affected.

The **File Menu** option allows you to enter information pertaining to the practice, change the date, and choose default data. It also allows you to back up and restore data and contains the File Maintenance option.

Set Program Date

This text contains a simulated work program, which will take you through many of the duties a medical billing specialist encounters in a given day. However, to make all data match properly, the entry dates for the data will need to be matched.

MediSoft is a date-sensitive program, and it is important when completing the exercises in this book to use the date that is provided. Many operations function using the date entered, such as the printing of day sheets and other reports. Throughout this text you will be given the date to use.

The Simulated Work Program starts at the beginning of the year so that you can see how deductibles and other items on a patient chart are accumulated. Thus, all initial data that is entered should use the date January 1 of the current year.

Every time you enter the MediSoft program you must be sure you are working on the correct date. Go through each of the following steps each time you begin working on the computer. As you enter the Simulated Work Program part of the course, you will encounter five different days. Be sure to reset the date as you begin each new day that is given in the program. If you do not, your data will not be recorded accurately, and your reports will not print properly.

Exercise **4-1**

Reset the date to January 14, CCYY by doing the following steps:

1. Click on the **File** Menu option.

2. Choose **Set Program Date** by either clicking on it or by striking **D** (the underlined letter).

3. Click on the (right/left arrows) next to the current month to move backward or forward through the months until you reach January, or click on the month shown and choose a month.

4. If the year is not correct, click on the year shown, and choose CCYY (with CCYY being replaced by the current year).

5. A January CCYY calendar will appear. Click on the **14** within the date boxes to indicate that this is January 14.

This will change the date for this use of the program. However, each time you exit the program then go back in, you will need to reset the date.

The current date that the computer believes it to be will be shown in the lower-right corner of the screen. You should glance at this date on a regular basis during this program to ensure that you are entering data on the correct date.

Note Regarding Dates

Please note that when YY is used in reference to a date, the YY indicates the current year (12/01/YY). When PY is used in reference to a date, the PY indicates the prior year (or last year) (12/01/PY). When NY is used in reference to a date, NY indicates the next year (12/01/NY).

New Practice/Open Practice

First we need to start by creating the practice we will be working with. MediSoft allows you to store a number of practices in different areas, thus allowing you to only work on the billing of one practice at a time and prevents the billing of separate providers from becoming mixed.

It is important to open the practice at the beginning of each session, or you will not be able to locate the patients, transactions, and other items that have been entered.

If you are doing billing for more than one practice (i.e., you work for a billing service that bills for numerous practices) it is important that you close one practice and open the correct practice before switching from one practice to another. If you do not do so, you may enter data into the wrong practice. To switch from one practice to another, click on **File**, then on **Open Practice**. Next, choose the specific practice you wish to work on.

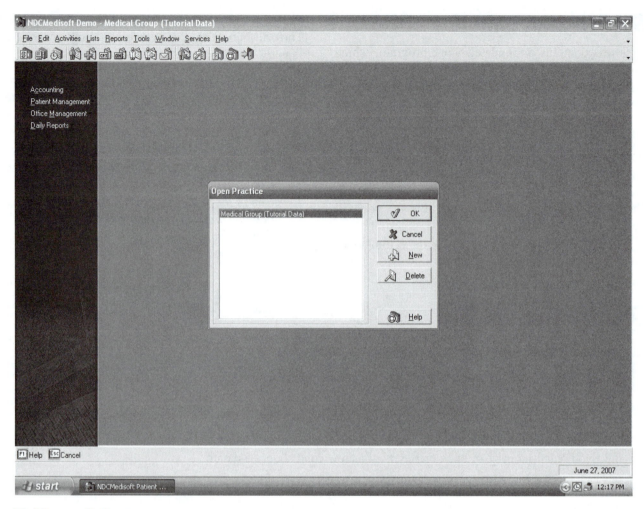

■ **Figure 4–1** Open Practice

Open Practice (**see Figure 4–1**) allows access to practices that have been previously entered. Once you have created the CHS practice, you will use the **Open Practice** option to access its information.

Practice Information/ Billing Service

The information contained in these screens will show up on various reports throughout the program, so it is important to ensure that the information is complete and correct.

Practice Information is where you enter information about the actual provider of services. Billing Service is where you enter information about the company that handles billing for that provider. Because CHS does its own billing, the billing information screen should be left blank.

Both the practice and billing information screens include the same fields. The information contained in these screens includes the following information:

Practice Name—The name of the office. If you are working for an individual provider, the provider's name may go in this field. You may enter up to 30 characters (either letters, punctuation, or spaces).

Street—The street address of the office or provider. You may enter up to 30 characters. If abbreviation is needed, be sure the information given on the line is sufficient to allow mail to be properly delivered.

A second street line has been created to allow you to enter additional data. This could be a suite number or a department to which items should be addressed (i.e., Billing Department).

Exercise 4-2

For this class, you will be working for Consolidated Health Services. To enter its practice information, click on the **File** menu option, and then choose **New Practice.** Enter "Consolidated Health Services," and choose a data path.

To prevent your data from being corrupted by others using MediSoft on your computer, the practice name and data path should include your name. For example: Practice: Consolidated Health Services Mary. Data Path: C:\MediSoft\CHSMary. Then click **Create**.

A **Practice Information (see Figure 4–2)** screen will open. As you read through the descriptions of the following fields, enter the following information on your screen. Entries and corrections are made by pressing Tab until you reach the field in which you wish to enter or change data. You may also use your mouse to position the arrow in the correct field and then click the left button. Once you have highlighted the field, type in the correct information and press Tab to move to the next field.

Enter the following information:

Practice Name: Consolidated Health Services
(your name)
Street: 1357 Castle Blvd.
Suite 515
City: Colter
State: CO
Zip Code: 81222
Phone: (790) 555-4567
Fax Phone: (790) 555-6789
Type: Medical
Federal Tax ID: 80-1234567

*When you have entered all data, be sure to save your changes by clicking on the **Save** box or by pressing **F3**. This will save the information to the database. Neglecting to do so will cause the data entered to be lost.*

City—The city of the provider/biller. You may enter up to 20 characters.

State—The state in which the provider/biller practices. This should coincide with the official postal two-letter state abbreviation. (See Appendix A for postal abbreviation codes).

Zip Code—The provider's/biller's zip code. If the complete nine-digit zip code is known, enter the first five digits, a hyphen, and the remaining four digits.

Phone—The provider's phone number. The area code and phone number should be entered without parentheses or hyphens separating the numbers. The computer will automatically enter these marks where needed.

Extension—The phone extension of the office.

Fax Phone—The provider's/biller's fax phone number. The area code and phone number should be entered without parentheses or hyphens separating the numbers. The computer will automatically enter these marks where needed.

Type—MediSoft can be used by medical practices, anesthesiologists, chiropractors, and many other healthcare providers. Choose Medical, Anesthesia, or Chiropractic. If you are billing for several types of practitioners, this field should be reset to reflect the types of claims you are currently entering. Choosing Anesthesia will allow anesthesia minutes to be entered onto claims. Choosing Chiropractic will add a field for "Level of Subluxation." Consolidated Health Services is a medical provider, so you should choose **Medical**. However, there may be a few times you need to enter anesthesia claims. At that time you should reset the practice type to Anesthesia.

Federal Tax ID—Enter the tax ID number for the practice. This can be either an employer identification

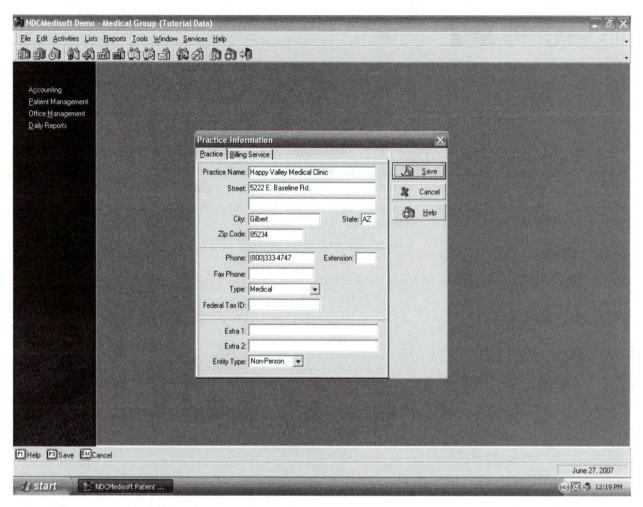

■ **Figure 4–2** Practice Information

number (EIN) for a business, or a social security number (SSN) for an individual provider practice. Because this number may take either form, hyphens should be entered in the appropriate places.

Extra 1:/Extra 2—These fields allow for entry of additional information that is important.

Program Options

A couple of program options should be checked before we proceed with the entry of codes, patients, and charges. These include a couple of the default settings that appear in the program.

1. Choose **File**.
2. Choose **Program Options (see Figure 4–3)**.

This brings up the program options, which have been entered. There are five pages of program options: General, Data Entry, Aging Reports, HIPAA (the Health Insurance Portability and Accountability Act of 1996), and Audit.

The **General** options include reminding you to back up your data before exiting the program and the windows, which will appear on the screen as you start up the program. We will not be changing the settings on this page.

To get to the Data Entry options, click on the **Data Entry** tab or press **E**.

You do want to use "**Enter to move between the fields**" and "**Force Payments To Be Applied**," so be sure there is a √ in the box to the left of these choices. These boxes are toggle (on/off) switches. Thus, clicking once on either the box or the words next to the box will turn the item on. Clicking it again will turn it off. The √ indicates the item is turned on.

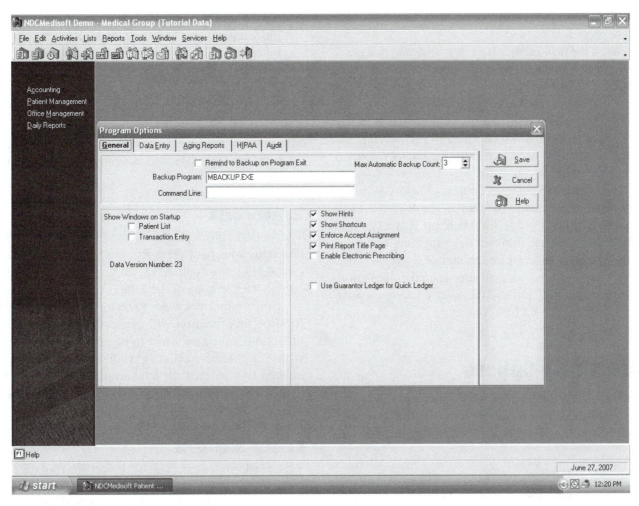

■ **Figure 4–3**   Program Options

You also want the computer to "Multiply units times amount," so be sure there is a √ in the box to the left of this choice. When entering transaction entries, it is possible to indicate that a procedure was performed several times or for several days by entering an appropriate number in the days or units field. A √ in this box will tell the computer to multiply the number of days or units by the charge for this service. Thus, if a doctor performs a minimal hospital visit on a patient two times over two days, the computer will show an extended charge of $200 total instead of the normal $100 per visit charge. **Default Place of Service:** Entering a location code in this field will automatically print this default code as the location of services on the Transaction Entry screen. These codes correspond to the two-digit place of service (location) codes used in item 24B of the 1500 Health Insurance Claim Form. The most common locations are

11	Office
21	Inpatient Hospital
22	Outpatient Hospital
23	Emergency Room

For a complete list of codes, see instructions for completing a 1500 Health Insurance Claim Form or the back of some 1500 Health Insurance Claim forms.

Once a default code is entered, it will appear on every transaction entry charge. If the default location code is incorrect for the service provided, it may be changed by simply typing in a new location code.

Because most of our billing will be for a medical office, we will use 11 as the default code.

To get to the Aging Reports options, click on the **Aging Reports** tab or press **A**.

Select the date and column parameters your office wishes to use when printing Patient or Insurance Aging Reports.

To get to the HIPAA options, click on the **HIPAA** tab or press **I**.

With the new privacy laws, it is essential that practices protect their data from unauthorized use or viewing. This function automatically logs off the program if there has been no activity for a set period of time. Basically, this option will shut off your computer if you stop using it or walk away from it. To get back into the program you will need to reenter the security code, if one is required for your office.

The Audit tab contains options to help you designate what information you want available in the Audit Generator. This topic is for MediSoft Advanced and MediSoft Network Professional programs only and should be left unaltered for this course.

Once you have entered the desired information, exit the Program Options Screen by clicking on **Save** or by pressing the **F3** function key.

Remaining Options

The remaining options on the File screen will not be used at this time. However, to familiarize you with their functions, please read the following information.

Backup Data

Backing up your files is a safety precaution that actually saves your data to a second file or to a disk. Then if one file has a problem, you have the information stored in a second place. MediSoft compresses the data at the time of backup to allow you to store more information on the files.

> **Destination Path**—Enter the file or drive that holds your backup disk. Be sure that your disks have been formatted and inserted in the appropriate drive before answering this question. It may take more than one disk to back up your files. If so, the MediSoft system will prompt you when to insert a new diskette. The screen will tell you how far along the backup process is. It is important not to shut off the computer during the backup process, as it could corrupt your data files.
>
> **Existing Backup Files**—This field will show you the backup files that currently exist on the data path or drive you have chosen. This helps prevent you from copying over backup files you may need.
>
> **Password**—If the security option requires that a password be entered to back up data, the password

would be entered here. Not all practices will require a password to back up data. However, using a password ensures that unauthorized persons are not able to make a copy of your patient files.

View Backup Disks

This option allows you to view the contents of a disk to be sure that the data was actually recorded to the backup disk.

Restore Data

This option allows you to restore (put back) information onto your hard drive that was either lost or corrupted. For this option to work, you must have a current backup copy of the data.

Be sure that you wish to restore the data, as performing this function will cause all MediSoft information on your hard drive to be erased and replaced with the MediSoft data on the data diskette or backup file. Insert your backup disk into the proper disk drive, and then follow the instructions on the screen.

Backup Root Data

This window is where you back up your root data directory, (i.e., C:\Medidata). The information backed up can include registration information and other files shared among all your practices.

Restore Root Data

This window is where you restore a backup of the root data directory. The information backed up can include registration information and other files shared among all your practices.

Security Setup

This option allows you to enter information on those people who are authorized to use the MediSoft system. It will also allow you to limit their access to certain files or commands.

File Maintenance

Choosing this option allows you to restore and rebuild your data files. This enables you to preserve the data and prevents you from having to reenter everything should a problem with your data files occur. Also included in this menu option is the ability to purge (erase) information and recalculate patient balances.

Rebuild Indexes

This option allows you to rebuild the index files when they become damaged. If index files are not damaged, this procedure is not necessary because MediSoft automatically maintains all index files. However, it is recommended that you rebuild all indexes prior to doing the month-end processing. This will ensure that all indexes are in a clean, undamaged state. Choose the index file(s) you wish to rebuild.

Rebuilding indexes can take a long time, depending on the amount of data contained in the indexes. Be sure to allow appropriate time. One of the best times to rebuild data indexes is to choose Rebuild All Files/ Indexes just prior to leaving work for the night. Interruptions (power failures or surges, etc.) will not cause irreparable damage as the old index files are not deleted until the rebuilding has been completed.

Pack Data

In MediSoft, as in many computer programs, information that has been deleted is not actually erased from the file. It is simply marked as deleted, and the computer reuses that space when it needs to by recording new data over the old. This is similar to recording over previous messages on an answering machine or tape recorder rather than erasing the messages and then taping a new message over the blank tape.

This option allows you to erase the deleted data, thus condensing the amount of data in your files and increasing the amount of free storage space on your disk. To use this option, choose the file(s) you wish to purge (erase) deleted data from.

You should back up your data prior to using this function, just in case data has been inadvertently deleted from the system. When ready to proceed, be sure you have enough available disk space to complete the operation.

Recalculate Balances

This option allows you to recalculate and update patient balances and reset the date and amount of the last payment made by each patient. Recalculating balances updates the patient reference balances. These balances are used on the ledger window, walkout receipts, day sheets, and superbills.

If you wish to recalculate a single patient's balance information, this can be done in the Transaction Screen by clicking on the Account Total amount.

Purge Data

This option allows you to erase data from your data files, thus condensing the amount of data in your files and increasing the amount of free storage space on your disk. To use this option, choose the file(s) you wish to purge (erase). Your choices include

- Appointment Purge
- Claim Purge
- Statement Purge
- Recall Purge
- Purge Closed Cases
- Credit Card Purge

To use this option, click on one of the preceding choices, and then enter a cutoff date (for the first four items). All data in that file before **and including** the date specified will be deleted. Thus, if you choose Appointment Purge and enter a date of 1/1/CCYY, all appointments that had been entered for dates prior to and including 1/1/CCYY will be deleted.

Before a claim can be deleted using this system, it must be marked "Done." Therefore, it must have been printed, billed, and paid (or adjusted out). Claims that have a remaining balance due will not be purged.

You also have the option of purging **all closed cases**. By selecting this option, all closed cases will be purged, regardless of whether there is an outstanding balance or not. (For further information on "cases," see Chapter 7 of this text.)

You can also purge **Credit Card Entries**. Only credit card entries that are inactive are purged from the program. All credit card entries that are purged are recorded in the audit file. Purging removes the credit card entry number from the transaction file.

You should back up your data prior to using this function, just in case data has been inadvertently deleted from the system. When ready to proceed, be sure you have enough available disk space to complete the operation.

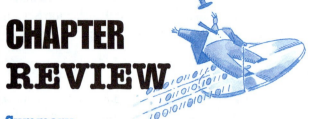

CHAPTER REVIEW

- The File Maintenance menu option allows you to rebuild your data files, recalculate balances, and purge data.

Summary

- The File Menu options allow you to enter information pertaining to the practice, change the date, and choose default data. It also allows you to back up and restore data, and contains the file Maintenance option.

Questions for Review

Directions: Answer the following questions without looking back into the material just covered. Write your answers in the space provided.

1. What is the importance of ensuring that the practice information is correct before performing any transactions?

_____

_____

_____

_____

_____

2. What three practice types are available in the Practice Information option screen?

1. _____

_____

2. _____

_____

3. _____

_____

3. What is the function of the Pack Data option?

_____

_____

_____

_____

_____

4. What is the function of the Restore Data option?

_____

_____

_____

5. What does it mean to Purge Data from your files?

_____

_____

_____

_____

_____

If you were unable to answer any of the questions, refer back to that section, and then fill in the answers.

5
Lists Menu Options

After completion of this chapter
you will be able to:

- Search for and delete an entry.
- Enter information in the Insurance Carrier List, Address List, Provider List, Referring Provider List, electronic data interchangeable/electronic

medial claims (EDI/EMC) Receivers List, Billing Code List, Procedure/Payment/Adjustment List, MultiLink List, and Diagnosis List.

Before you can enter transactions and create claims you will need to enter some basic data into the computer. This data includes CPT® and ICD-9-CM codes, patient and insurance information, MultiLink codes, addresses, and provider information. Because many of the other lists are accessed when entering patient data (Patients/Guarantors and Cases), we will discuss the completion of the other screens first. Completing the patient data screens will be discussed in Chapter 6.

Searching for an Entry

When entering most of the following screens, you will be automatically brought into the search screen. A listing of the previously entered entities (insurance carriers, addresses, providers, etc.) will appear in the middle of the screen. Highlight (click on) the entry you wish to access, and then choose Edit at the bottom of the screen.

If the entity you wish to work on is not shown in the search screen, you must search for it. To search for a specific entry, first choose whether you wish to look for it under the code listing or by name. Different lists may have additional search options, for example, description, type, and so on. Make this selection in the **Field:** field by clicking on the "down arrow" on the top-right side of the screen. It is usually easiest to sort by name because the code is not always known. To specify your preferred search parameters, click on the magnifying glass icon or down arrow (↓) to the right of the **Search for:** field.

As you enter a code or name in the **Search for:** field, the list in the lower part of the screen will automatically show all matching records. The more characters entered into the field, the more specific and narrow your search results will be. If there are no matches, the list will be blank. If there are several matches, you will be given a list of choices. Highlight the appropriate choice by clicking on it and clicking Edit. That entity's name and information will then appear on the screen.

To conduct a search in previous versions of MediSoft, click on the ↓ to the right of the **Sort By:** field. This will bring up the choice of sorting by code or by name.

Then move the cursor to the search field by clicking on the box to the right of Search. Enter a portion of the entity's name (i.e., Bal for Ball Insurance), then press enter. If there are no matches, you will hear a beep. If there is only one match, that entity's information will appear on the screen. If there are several matches, you will be given a list of choices. Click on the appropriate choice and press enter. That entity's name and information will then appear on the screen.

If you wish to enter a new entity, click on the "New" box at the bottom of the screen, or press **F8**.

Deleting an Entry

To delete an entity from any of the following lists, search for the entity using the search screen. Once found, highlight the entity's name on the screen, then hit the Delete key, or click on the Delete box at the bottom of the screen. You will be asked: "Are you sure you want to delete this record?" If so, click on "Yes," and the record will be deleted.

EDI/EMC Receivers List

Because information in the EDI/EMC Receivers List is used in several of the remaining lists, we will discuss it first.

With today's new technology, providers have the ability to transmit claims from their computers through phone lines and directly into another computer. This is called electronic data interchange (EDI). In earlier versions of MediSoft, claims sent in this manner are called electronic media claims (EMC). Claims printed on paper and sent through the regular mail system are often called paper claims.

Electronic versus Paper Claims

Electronic media claims have certain advantages over paper claims:

1. They take less time to submit because they are transmitted directly through phone lines. There is no need to wait several days for them to be sent through the mail.
2. They use less paper and other supplies.
3. There is less of a chance that they will be lost or misplaced.
4. They are processed much more quickly (an average of about 10 to 15 days, rather than the normal 30 days for paper claims).
5. There is less chance for error because the information does not need to be reentered into the insurance carrier's computer.
6. There is less chance of the claim being rejected because it often goes through a clearinghouse, which will do a preliminary check to make sure all required fields are completed.
7. It lowers costs, requiring less personnel time for printing and mailing the claims and for entering the data in the insurance carrier computers.
8. It saves time for the provider because each claim does not need to be signed. The provider's signature on the agreement between the insurance carrier and the provider is considered valid for all claims submitted electronically.

Direct Submission versus Clearinghouse

When claims are submitted electronically, they are sent through the phone lines using a modem. Some carriers allow you to submit claims directly to them, but many others prefer that the claims first be sent to a clearinghouse. The clearinghouse then checks the claims to be sure that all the necessary information has been completed on the claim and there are no glaring errors (i.e., female procedure performed on a male patient, procedures with no relationship to the given diagnosis, etc.). Once checked, the claims are then sent on to the insurance carrier.

Using a clearinghouse allows the carrier to reject fewer claims because those that are not complete or have glaring errors are never submitted to them. It saves personnel time as well as resources that might be spent contacting the provider for further information. Be sure to follow HIPAA guidelines when submitting claims.

Submitting Claims Using MediSoft

The MediSoft system allows you to submit claims electronically either through a clearinghouse or directly to a carrier. Once all the data has been entered through the appropriate screens, claims can be generated and sent using the Claim Management screen.

Training facilities cannot submit electronic claims because they have not been assigned appropriate clearinghouse codes, and to go through the process of submitting a claim electronically would actually send the claim out. Additionally, trying to send out claims when your computer is not properly hooked up to phone lines could cause some of your data to be lost. For that reason, CHS will submit all claims on paper. However, a preliminary relationship with a clearinghouse has been established, so we will enter the data we currently have on them.

The first step to creating electronic data interchange/electronic media claims is to enter the information regarding the company that will be receiving the claims. This can be either the insurance carrier directly or a clearinghouse.

Exercise 5-1

CHS will be submitting claims through a clearinghouse. In the Lists menu, click on EDI/EMC Receivers. At the bottom of the screen, click New. Enter the following information for the clearinghouse:

Name: EDI Always
Address: 4123 Media Blvd.
Colter, CO 81225
Phone: (800) 555-3452 X456
Fax: (800) 555-6789
Contact: Emily Encoder
Data Phone: (800) 555-3746
Submitter ID: CHSAA123
Password: CHS0001

There are three screens in the EDI/EMC Receiver List: the Address, Modem, and ID and Extra screens.

Address Screen

Code—The computer will automatically assign an access code for each address entered, or you can enter a code yourself. Codes may contain letters or numbers and can be up to five characters.

Name—Enter the name of the EDI/EMC receiving company. You have up to 30 characters.

Street—Enter the street address of the EDI/EMC receiving company. Two lines are provided to allow for a complete address.

City—Enter the city of the EDI/EMC receiving company.

State—Enter the state of the EDI/EMC receiving company. This should correspond with the two-letter postal code for a state.

Zip Code—Enter the zip code of the EDI/EMC receiving company. If the complete nine-digit zip code is known, enter the first five digits, a hyphen, and the remaining four digits.

Phone—Enter the EDI/EMC receiving company's phone number. This should be the number you can call and reach a person, not the number that your computer/modem should call to connect with their computer/modem. No hyphens or parentheses are needed. The computer will automatically enter these.

Fax—Enter the EDI/EMC receiving company's fax number. No hyphens or parentheses are needed. The computer will automatically enter these.

Contact—Enter your contact within the EDI/EMC receiving company. This can be either a person or a department.

Comment—Enter any comments regarding the EDI/EMC receiving company. These can be items such as the best time to call them, their hours, or other pertinent information.

Modem Screen

Data Phone—Enter the phone number that your modem should call to reach their modem. This is often different from the regular phone number.

Dialing Prefix—Enter any prefix needed for dialing this number. If this is an international number, enter the country code.

Dialing Suffix—Enter any suffix needed for dialing this number.

Serial Port/Parity/Baud Rate/Data Bits/Transmit Protocol/Stop Bits—This is information detailing the type of modem you have and how it sends information (speed, etc.). This information should appear automatically if your computer is already connected to a modem. If not, you will need to consult the manual for your specific type of modem for the correct data to enter here.

Modem Initialization—This field is normally left blank. It is used only when you are having difficulties with the program not "hanging up" after the transmission. You may also need this option if the modem is required to be left in a certain state (i.e., Auto Answer mode).

Modem Termination—Some modems require a string of characters to notify the modem that the transmission is complete and the call should be terminated. Your modem instruction manual will tell you if this applies to your modem. In most cases, this field is left blank.

Dialing Attempt—Enter the number of attempts you want your computer to make before abandon-

ing the attempt to send information. If this field is left blank, the program will make up to 99 dialing attempts.

Transmission Mode—You have two choices for this setting. Test is used if you are not actively sending a claim, but merely want to test if the EDI/EMC receiver is properly receiving your transmission. Active is used if you are actually sending a claim. For this class, this field should always be set to Test.

ID and Extra Screen

Submitter ID 1 and 2—This is a code that will be given to the practice by the EDI/EMC receiver. It allows the EDI/EMC receiver to identify who is sending the claims. It is similar to an account number. MediSoft allows up to two submitter IDs for each EDI/EMC receiver.

Submitter Password 1 and 2—This field is for entering the password to submit claims. This is similar to having a password at the bank before your account can be accessed. It is a security precaution to ensure that others do not submit claims using your account number because clearinghouses often charge by the number of claims submitted.

Program File—This is a number given to you by your EDI/EMC receiver.

Extra 1 through 6—These fields are for entering additional data that is needed to submit claims to this EDI/EMC receiver. The data to be entered in these fields will often be assigned by the EDI/EMC receiver.

File Name ID—This is a field that allows MediSoft to communicate by modem with the MediSoft clearinghouse. This field should not be changed unless you are instructed to do so by MediSoft.

Be sure to save your data before exiting this screen.

Insurance Carrier List

To access the Insurance Carrier List (**see Figure 5–1**) click on the Insurance Carrier List icon, or choose the **Lists** Menu option and choose **Insurance Carriers**.

This option allows you to see and enter information regarding a patient's insurance carrier. This includes not only the name and address for the insurance carrier,

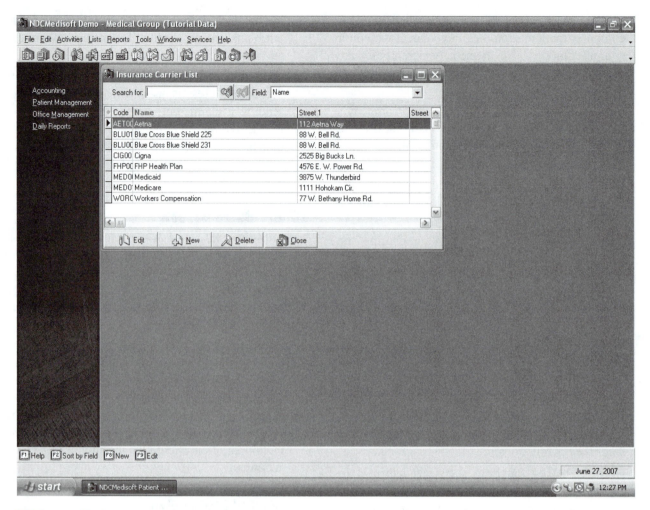

■ **Figure 5–1**   Insurance Carrier List

but also the insurance type and information on how the carrier prefers to have forms printed.

To enter a new insurance carrier, click New at the bottom of the screen or press the **F8** function key. To edit the information of an insurance carrier that is already entered, click on the carrier in the list and click Edit at the bottom of the screen or press the **F9** function key.

When creating or editing insurance carrier information, you will input information into various screens. The MediSoft Patient Accounting Program includes Address, Options, EDI Codes, and PINs screens. Earlier versions of the software have only Address, Options, and EMC Codes screens.

Exercise 5-2

Sue Pervisor gives you the patient information sheet for the Dunnit family (Document 5 from Section 4). While going through the instructions for this screen, enter the insurance carrier data for this family.

Address Screen

The address screen allows you to enter name, address, and phone information of an insurance carrier.

Code—The computer will automatically assign a code for each carrier entered. If desired,

you may assign a code. This can be a series of numbers or letters. Some practices will choose to enter the first five characters of the insurance carrier's name. If those numbers have already been used, then enter the first four characters followed by a number (i.e., Winter Insurance would be Winte, Wintell Insurers would be Wint1, etc.).

Name—Enter the name of the insurance carrier. This field must be completed or you will not be allowed to save this carrier.

Street—Enter the street address of the insurance carrier. You have two lines to enter their complete address. If mail is to be addressed to a specific department (i.e., Attn: Claims Dept.), that information can be placed on the first line with the street address given on the following line.

City—Enter the city in which the insurance carrier is located.

State—Enter the state in which the insurance carrier is located. This should coincide with the official postal two-letter state abbreviation.

Zip Code—Enter the insurance carrier's zip code. If the complete nine-digit zip code is known, enter the first five digits, a hyphen, and the remaining four digits.

Phone—Enter the insurance carrier's phone number. Do not add hyphens or parentheses; the computer will automatically put these in.

Extension—Enter the extension for the insurance carrier. This will often be the extension for the claims department because they are the department that is most often contacted by a provider.

Fax—Enter the insurance carrier's fax phone number. Do not add hyphens or parentheses.

Contact—Enter the name of your contact at the insurance carrier, if known. This can be a specific person who handles your accounts or the name of a department.

Practice ID Number—Many insurance carriers, especially HMOs and PPOs, assign a number to the practice to help identify it. If applicable, enter that number here.

Options Screen

To get to the Options screen, simply click on the word **Options** at the top of the Insurance Carrier List screen.

Plan Name—Enter the plan name assigned by the insurance carrier. This allows the insurance carrier to more readily access the proper contract or policy. This information corresponds with box 9d or 11c on a 1500 Health Insurance Claim form.

Type—This item will indicate the type of claim being submitted to this carrier. Click on the ↓

arrow to the right of the Type: field to bring up a complete list of insurance carrier types. To choose a type, simply click on the type desired.

Q1. Bring up the list of insurance carrier types, and then look at a 1500 Health Insurance Claim form. If one of the first seven Type codes is chosen, where will this information show up on a 1500 Health Insurance Claim form?

Procedure Code Set—It is possible to enter up to three procedure codes for a given procedure. This is most often used with Medicare Healthcare Common Procedure Coding System (HCPCS) codes and with states or carriers that have their own coding system. The Current Procedural Terminology (CPT®) code should be entered in the first procedure code box, then the corresponding HCPCS or state procedure code entered into the second and third code fields. By entering a 1, 2, or 3, MediSoft knows which set of codes to use when billing this carrier. For this class, if no code set is indicated on your paperwork, enter 1 to print CPT® codes. If this is for a Medicare claim, enter 2 to indicate the use of HCPCS codes.

Diagnosis Code Set—Likewise, it is possible to enter up to three diagnosis codes for a given diagnosis. This is most often used with states or carriers that have their own coding system. The *International Classification of Diseases,* Ninth Edition (ICD-9) code should be entered in the first diagnosis code box, then the corresponding state diagnosis code entered into the second and third code fields. By entering a 1, 2, or 3, MediSoft knows which set of codes to use when billing this carrier. For this class, enter 1 to print ICD-9-CM codes.

Patient Signature on File/Insured Signature on File/Physician Signature on File—Different carriers occasionally prefer to have different items printed in the signature boxes of the 1500 Health Insurance Claim form (items 12, 13, and 31). Click on the ↓ to the right of each Signature on File field. If this carrier wishes the words "Signature on File" to print in the 1500 Health Insurance Claim form signature boxes, click on that option. To print the name of the patient and/or insured in items 12 and 13 and the name of the provider in item 31, click on the Print Name option. If you wish nothing to print in items 12, 13, and 31, click on Leave Blank. If nothing is printed in the boxes, the patient will need to sign items 12 and 13, and the provider will need to sign item 31 before the claim can be submitted.

Although these boxes will determine what the carrier wishes to have printed in the box ("Signature on File," the patient's/insured's/physician's name, or nothing), the patient and the physician have the right to determine whether or not they agree to the provisions listed in these boxes. The patient must have previously signed an authorization to release information and an assignment of benefits. If these documents are not signed, then nothing should be printed in these boxes. For that reason, the patient information file in the Patient/Guarantor List (see Chapter 6) has a box to indicate whether or not these items have been signed. Therefore, the patient record actually controls whether anything will be placed in these boxes. This box only allows the carrier to determine what wording they prefer to have written in these boxes if the permission has been granted.

Likewise, the provider information screen in the Provider List allows the provider to make the determination of whether the computer will sign the form for him (using "Signature on File" or the provider's name) or whether the item will be left blank.

For this class, all insurance carriers should have nothing placed in the signature boxes. The biller should sign each 1500 Health Insurance Claim form as the provider representative.

Print PINs on Forms—Occasionally, services rendered in a provider's office will be rendered by staff other than the provider. Medicare and Medicaid require that, if the provider rendering services is not the attending provider (the one listed in item 33 of the 1500 Health Insurance Claim form), that the provider who rendered each service be identified in box 24K of the 1500 Health Insurance Claim form.

This box allows you the option of printing the provider's name and PIN, printing the PIN only, or leaving the area blank. For this class, leave the area blank.

Default Billing Method—This box allows you to choose whether this carrier prefers to have claims submitted electronically or on paper. By clicking on the ↓ to the right of this field, you can choose either Paper or Electronic. For this class, we will be printing all claims on paper. If a carrier

has agreed to accept electronic claims from this provider, choosing Electronic in this box will instruct the computer not to print these claims on paper, but to send them electronically.

EDI/EMC Codes Screen

The third screen is for entering information for submitting electronic media claims (EMC) to this carrier.

EDI/EMC Receiver—Enter the code for the EDI/EMC receiver (the company or organization that will receive your EDI/EMC claims for this carrier). For an EDI/EMC carrier to have a code, they must have previously been entered under the EDI/EMC Receivers List (see **List**, **EDI/EMC Receivers**). You may search for an EDI/EMC receiver's code by clicking on the magnifying glass to the right of this field or by pressing **F6**. If the EDI/EMC Receiver has not been previously entered, press **F8** to add it to the EDI/EMC Receiver List.

EDI/EMC Payor/EDI/EMC Sub-ID/NDC Record Code—These entry fields will be assigned to you by the Electronic Claims Submission company that handles your claims. They are used for identification purposes.

EDI/EMC Extra 1/Medigap/EDI/EMC Extra 2— These fields are for entering extra information regarding EDI/EMC claims for this carrier. They are often not used.

EDI Max Transactions—Some carriers will limit the number of claims that can be submitted at one time. Enter the maximum number of claims allowed by each carrier. Often this field is left blank.

After entering insurance carrier data, be sure to hit **F3** to save, or click on the **Save** button. The insurance carrier will then be added to the Insurance Carrier List, which will appear on the screen.

To exit the insurance carrier screen, click on the **Close** button.

Address List

This section of the MediSoft system is used as an address file to hold the names, addresses, and phone numbers that your practice needs. The MediSoft system also uses this section to store data

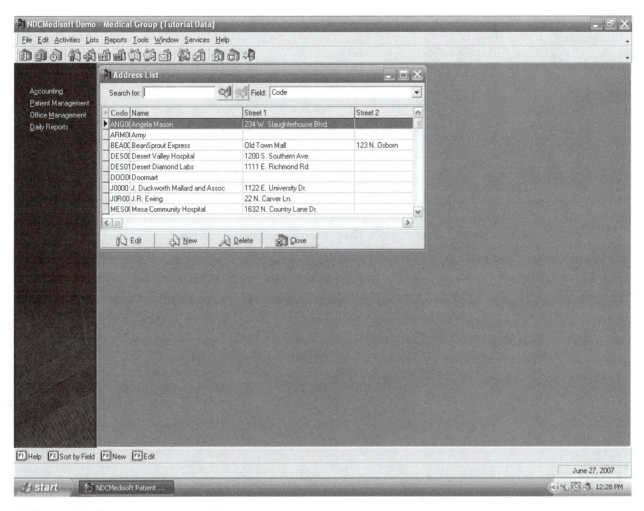

■ Figure 5–2   Address List

on a patient's employer. Other pertinent addresses may include referring physicians, facilities, or attorneys.

To access the **Address List (see Figure 5–2)**, click on the Address List icon, or choose the **Lists** Menu option and click **Addresses**.

Exercise 5-3

While reading through this screen, enter the pertinent information regarding place of employment for D. Jobb Dunnitt (Document 5). Click **New** to enter information.

Code: The computer will automatically assign an access number for each address entered, or you can enter a code yourself. Codes may contain letters or numbers and can be up to five characters.

Name: Enter the name of the person, employer, facility, etc.

Street: Enter the street address for the addressee.

City: Enter the city for the addressee.

State: Enter the state for the addressee. This should coincide with the official postal two-letter state abbreviation.

Zip Code: Enter the addressee's zip code. If the complete nine-digit zip code is known, enter the first five digits, a hyphen, and the remaining four digits.

Type: This field allows you to differentiate between the types of addresses listed. MediSoft has six types of address records:

- Attorney
- Employer
- Facility*
- Laboratory
- Miscellaneous
- Referral Source.

*A facility address can be any type of medical facility, including a hospital, urgent care facility, rest home, and so forth.

Phone: Enter the addressee's phone number. Do not use parentheses or hyphens.

Extension: Enter the extension for the addressee.

Fax Phone: Enter the addressee's fax phone number. Do not use parentheses or hyphens.

Cell Phone: Enter the addressee's personal cell phone number. Do not use parentheses or hyphens.

Office: Enter the addressee's office number, or the number at which he or she can be reached at work. Do not use parentheses or hyphens.

Contact: Enter the name of the contact person for the addressee if one is known.

E-Mail: Enter the addressee's e-mail address.

ID: Enter the Unique Physician Identification Number (UPIN) for referring providers. This number will then print in the required box on the 1500 Health Insurance Claim form (item 17a).

Identifier: Enter the Employer Identification Number (EIN) for the addressee. This is a HIPAA-compliance field.

Extra 1/Extra 2: Enter additional data regarding the person or entity listed.

Provider List

This screen is for entering information about the providers in the practice. Additional practice staff (i.e., nurses, billers) may also be entered in this file.

To access the **Provider List (see Figure 5–3)**, click on the Provider List icon, or choose the **Lists** Menu option and choose **Providers**.

Exercise 5-4

Because the MediSoft system is new to CHS, none of the providers have been entered into the system. Take out the Provider Information List (Document 2). While going through the following descriptions, enter the information for the CHS doctors.

There are four information screens in the Provider List: Address, Default PINs, Default Group IDs, and PINs. In earlier versions there are just two screens in the Provider List: the Address screen and the PINs and IDs screen.

Address Screen

Code—The computer will automatically assign an access code for each provider entered, or you can enter a code yourself. Codes may contain letters or numbers and can be up to five characters. Up to 99 providers may be entered in this file.

(NOTE: If MediSoft assigns the code, it will often use the provider's initials.) Once a code has been assigned, it may not be changed.

Inactive—Check this box if you need to deactivate a provider, but not delete him/her. This may need to be done if a provider is no longer with the practice,

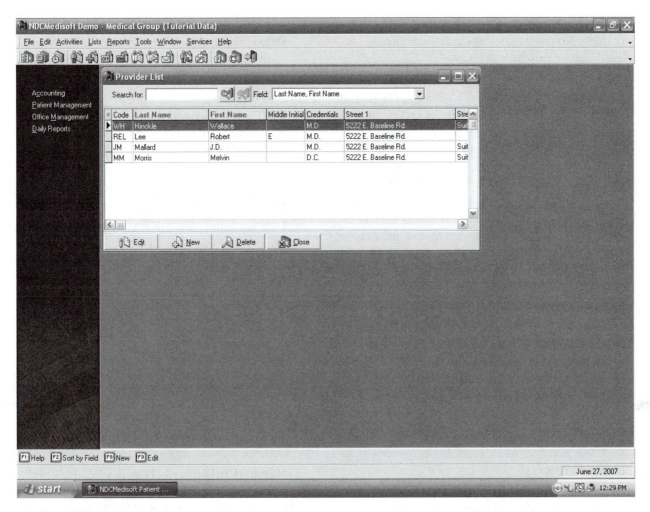

■ Figure 5–3   Provider List

but all the claims have not yet been paid. If there are still open issues on the claims of this provider, the provider needs to remain in the system. Placing a provider on inactive status may prevent you from entering new claims for this provider.

Last Name—Enter the last name of the provider. You have up to 20 characters. If the name is longer than 20 characters, most providers will prefer you to type in the name as it appears, until you run out of space. This will allow names to be alphabetized more correctly than if you attempt to abbreviate the name by leaving out letters in the middle of the name.

Middle Initial—Enter the middle initial of the provider.

First Name—Enter the first name of the provider.

Credentials—Enter the provider's credentials. This will normally be M.D.

Street—Enter the street address of the provider. Two lines are provided to allow for a complete address.

City—Enter the provider's city.

State—Enter the provider's state. This should correspond with the two-letter postal code for a state.

Zip Code—Enter the provider's zip code. If the complete nine-digit zip code is known, enter the first five digits, a hyphen, and the remaining four digits.

E-Mail—Enter the provider's e-mail address.

Office—Enter the provider's office phone number. No hyphens or parentheses are needed.

Fax—Enter the provider's fax number. No hyphens or parentheses are needed.

Home—Enter the provider's home phone number. No hyphens or parentheses are needed.

Cell—Enter the provider's personal cell phone number. No parentheses or hyphens are needed.

Signature on File—This box determines whether the computer will print "Signature on File" or the physician's name in item 31 of the 1500 Health Insurance Claim form. This is an on/off choice. By clicking on this option, it will place an X in the box if there is not one or remove the X if there is one. If an X is placed in the box, the Signature Date field will be highlighted to allow you to enter the date on which the provider's signature was placed on file. CHS requires all claims to be signed by the provider or the provider's representative (you). Therefore nothing should be printed in this field. You should sign and date all claims.

Medicare Participating—Many providers sign agreements with Medicare for treating Medicare patients. Among other things, this agreement limits the amount that the provider can accept for payment of services to Medicare patients. If the provider accepts Medicare assignment, enter an X in this box. If not, leave it blank.

License Number—Each state licenses providers to practice in that state. Enter the provider's state license number.

Specialty—Indicate the provider's specialty. For a complete list of specialties, click on the ↓ to the right of the field. Then choose a specialty by clicking on the appropriate specialty for the provider.

Default PINs Screen

SSN/Federal Tax ID—All persons and companies are required to have a tax ID number. For individuals, this is a Social Security Number (SSN). For companies, it is an employer identification number (EIN). Enter the tax ID number here, including hyphens in the appropriate places, and indicate whether this is an SSN or EIN in the toggle boxes to the right.

Medicare PIN—This field is for a single provider's Medicare assigned PIN.

Medicaid PIN/Medicare PIN/Blue Cross/Blue Shield PIN/Commercial PPO/HMO PIN—Medicaid, TRICARE/CHAMPUS, Blue Cross/Blue Shield, and some other commercial carriers may also use identifying numbers for their providers. Enter each that applies in the appropriate fields. When any of these fields, the Provider

Identification Number (PIN) field or the Unique Physician Identification Number (UPIN) field, are used, the computer will print the appropriate PIN number in item 33 of the 1500 Health Insurance Claim form.

PPO—If the provider is a member of a preferred provider organization (PPO) network, enter the assigned PPO number here.

HMO—If the provider is a member of a health maintenance organization (HMO) network, enter the assigned HMO number here.

UPIN—Enter the provider's Unique Physician Identifying Number (UPIN). When a provider orders services for a Medicare patient or refers a patient to another provider, this number is required.

Q2. Where does a referring provider's UPIN appear on a 1500 Health Insurance Claim form?

EDI/EMC ID—Providers are often assigned an identifying number for electronic media claims (EMC). This number would be assigned by the EMC clearinghouse. We will not be using this number.

National Identifier—This is a 15-digit alphanumeric identifier assigned by the Health Care Financing Administration (HCFA) now known as CMS. It is required for HIPAA compliance.

CLIA Number—The Clinical Laboratory Improvement Amendments (CLIA) number is assigned to lab providers submitting electronic claims through NDC.

TAT Number—This number is assigned to providers submitting electronic claims through the National Drug Code (NDC).

Extra 1/Extra 2—Enter additional data regarding the person or entity listed earlier.

Default Group IDs Screen

Group Number—Often a provider is part of a medical group. In such a case, Medicare may assign a group Provider Identification Number (PIN) rather than one PIN to each of the doctors. If this is the case, enter the group PIN number here. All CHS doctors have the same group PIN. It is CHS123.

Medicare Group ID—If the group has a Medicare assigned UPIN, enter that number here.

Medicaid Group ID—If the group has a Medicaid assigned UPIN, enter that number here.

BC/BS Group ID—If the group has a Blue Cross/Blue Shield assigned UPIN, enter that number here.

Other Group ID—If the group has any other assigned UPIN, enter that number here.

Q3. Where does a provider's group number appear on a 1500 Health Insurance Claim form?

PINs Screen

This screen shows a list of entered providers' PINs and Group IDs for the various insurance carriers they interact with and their corresponding codes.

After entering each provider's data, be sure to hit **F3** to save, or click on the **Save** button. The provider will then be added to the Provider List.

To exit the Provider screen, click on the **Close** button.

Referring Provider List

The **Referring Provider List (see Figure 5–4)** is used for entering data on providers who have referred patients to the practice. It is used to track referrals and to complete Items 17 and 17a on the 1500 Health Insurance Claim form.

These fields are the same as the fields for the Provider List. For instructions on completing these fields, see prior information for Provider List.

Billing Code List

Often practices split their billing into several groups. This allows for continuous income during the month, as well as prevents the major backlog of work that can happen with billing all patients at once. By using this field, you can place patients into groups for billing purposes. Patients can be grouped together by last name (i.e., A–M is billed on the first of the month and N–Z

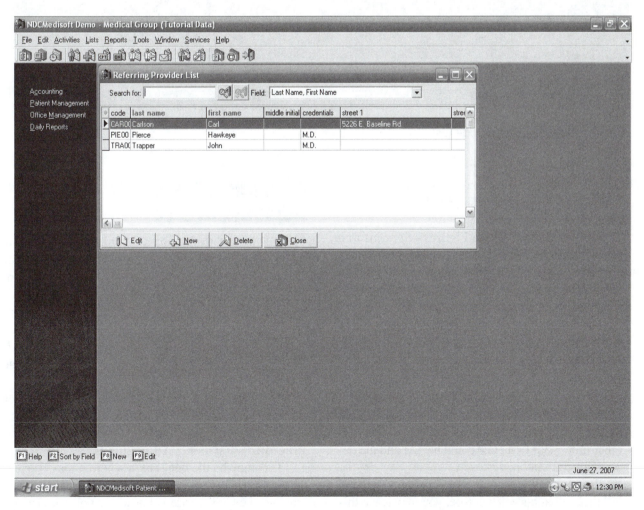

■ **Figure 5–4**   Referring Provider List

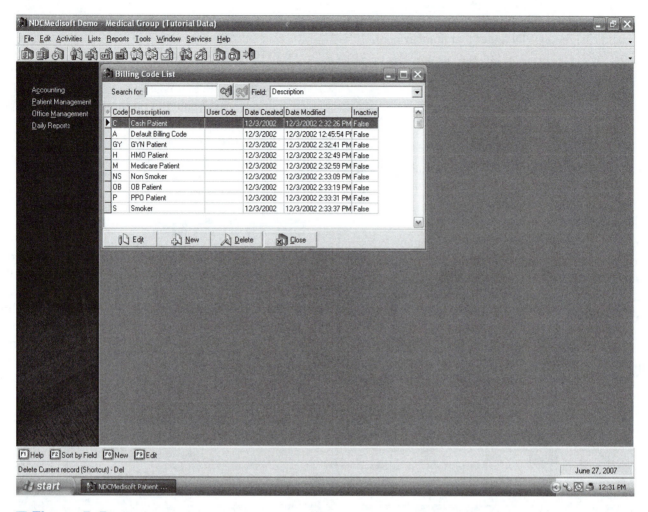

■ **Figure 5–5**   Billing Code List

is billed on the 15th of the month), insurance carrier or type of insurance (i.e., Medicare, Medicaid, group insurance), or by various other methods.

The Billing Code List (**see Figure 5–5**) opens to a window with a list alphabetized by code of all previously entered billing codes. From this window you can search for existing information. To enter new codes click **New** at the bottom of the window.

Code—A two-digit alphanumeric code, which identifies this billing code.

Description—A description of the billing code. For example, if you were to bill all patients with last names starting with A–M at one time, and all patients with last names starting with N–Z at another time, your first code could be AM and the description Patient Names A–M.

Because we are using so few patients, we will bill them all at once. Therefore, you may leave this space blank.

Procedure/Payment/Adjustment List

This file is used to store data regarding all transactions that may be used in the Transaction Entry screen. These include not only CPT® codes, but also payments and adjustments that are necessary for keeping accurate accounting records. In reality, many providers purchase computerized CPT® lists that can be automatically loaded into the computer each year. The practice then adds its own codes for payments and adjustments.

To access the Procedure/Payment/Adjustment List, (**see Figure 5–6**) click on the CPT® icon, or choose the **Lists** menu option and choose **Procedures/Payments/Adjustments**.

This may be the one screen where it may be easier to sort by the code rather than the description, based on whether the CPT® code is known or not. Descriptions of medical terms can sometimes be confusing, and

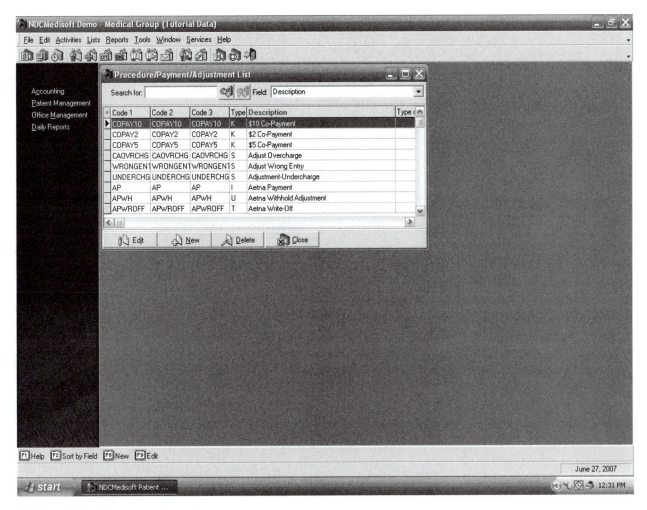

■ **Figure 5–6**   Procedure/Payment/Adjustment List

there are often numerous choices for the same type of procedure. For example, if you are searching for an office visit, you may end up with over 10 choices, depending on whether the patient is new or established and the complexity of the visit.

Exercise 5-5

Sue Pervisor gives you a list of procedures that have not yet been entered in the Procedure Code List (Document 3). Look up the proper procedure code in the CPT® and enter the procedures into the Procedure/Payment/Adjustment screen. All items are charges, and the accounting code should be given as 4010 for medicine charges, 4020 for surgery, 4030 for consultation, 4040 for diagnostic x-ray, 4050 for diagnostic lab, 4060 for radiation therapy, and 4070 for anesthesia.

When editing or creating new codes, there are two screens in the Procedure/Payment/Adjustment list; the General screen and the Amounts screen. The General screen provides all the necessary information regarding the type of code, the description, and insurance printing information. The Amounts screen contains information regarding the charges for the procedure and the cost to the practice.

General Screen

Code 1—Enter the procedure code. This can be either an alphabetical or numerical code of up to 10 characters. For CPT® codes, enter the five-digit CPT® code. Alphabetic codes would be entered for other procedures. For example, to indicate a cash payment by the patient, you could enter the code: CSHPMT.

Inactive—Check this box if you need to deactivate a code, but not delete it. This may need to be done if the American Medical Association (AMA) has deleted a CPT® code, but all previous claims with this code have not yet been paid. If there are still open issues on the claims, the code needs to remain in the system. Having a code on an inactive status may prevent you from entering this code on new claims.

Description—Enter a description of the procedure. Your entry space is limited. You are allowed up to 40 characters. When entering CPT® codes, be sure that all necessary information for choosing the correct CPT® code is entered in the description.

Q4. How would you abbreviate the following description: Office or outpatient visit with a problem-focused history and exam and straightforward medical decision making?

Write your description in the space provided. Do not use more than 40 characters.

_____

_____

_____

_____

Code Type—The following is an alphabetized list of the code types that may be present, depending on your version of the MediSoft software. You must choose one of the following code types to identify the type of procedure.

Adjustment—This code is used for adjustments to a charge. These can be anything such as a courtesy reduction of a patient's bill or a correction of an incorrect billing.

Billing Charge—These are normal charges used for billing.

Cash Copayment—If the patient pays his or her copayment by cash, this code should be used.

Cash Payment—The patient has made a cash payment on this account. This is for patients who make a cash payment on the amount of the charges that are their responsibility.

Check Copayment—If the patient pays his or her copayment by check, this code should be used.

Check Payment—This code indicates that a patient has paid for services with a personal check.

Comment—This code allows a comment to be entered onto the patient's account.

Credit Card Copayment—If the patient pays his or her copayment by credit card, this code should be used.

Credit Card Payment—If the patient made a payment by credit card, this code should be used.

Deductible—Indicates that this is a payment made to cover the patient's deductible amount.

Inside Lab Charge—If there were charges for a lab contained within the facility, this code should be used.

Insurance Adjustment—The amount has been adjusted due to information from the insurance carrier.

Insurance Payment—The insurance carrier is making a payment on this account.

Insurance Take Back Adjustment—An adjustment made by an insurance carrier.

Insurance Withhold Adjustment—An amount withheld by an insurance carrier until the end of the year. This amount must be adjusted against the patient's account.

Medicare Adjustment— This adjustment is being made to write off the difference between a billed charge and a Medicare-approved amount.

Outside Lab Charge— The charges are for a lab not connected with this facility.

Procedure Charge—The service being performed will create a charge on the patient's account. A charge code would be used for all CPT® codes and other services or procedures for which a patient is charged (i.e., missed appointment charge).

Product Charge—The charge is for a product rather than a procedure. For example, a person may require crutches to assist with walking or a sling for a sprained wrist.

Tax—The charges are for tax. This is usually associated with a product charge.

The practice may type in any code they wish to indicate services, charges, adjustments, etc., for any of these procedures. For example, an entry with the code MCRADJ and the code type of Adjustment could be used to identify the amount above the Medicare-approved amount that is being written off the patient's account. The practice may set up any number of procedure codes within a procedure type. Therefore, they can list several different types of adjustments, all with the Adjustment procedure type.

Account Code—Enter the four-digit general ledger account number that pertains to these services. This allows transactions to be categorized according to their type so that all similar charges, payments, or adjustments may be grouped together on reports and in the company's accounting system.

Type of Service—A complete list of these codes will be provided by your carrier. These codes correspond to the general descriptions given in the CPT® and add in a few other types of services. A partial list includes

1. —Medicine
2. —Surgery
3. —Consultation
4. —Diagnostic X-ray
5. —Diagnostic Lab
6. —Radiation Therapy
7. —Anesthesia
8. —Surgical Assistance
9. —Other Medical
0. —Blood Charges

Place of Service—Enter the two-digit code corresponding with the place where this service is normally performed (i.e., office visits are done in an office).

These codes correspond to the two-digit place of service (location) codes used in item 24B of the 1500 Health Insurance Claim form. The most common locations associated with medical billing are

11 Office
21 Inpatient Hospital
22 Outpatient Hospital
23 Emergency Room

For a complete list of codes, see instructions for completing a 1500 Health Insurance Claim form or the back of the many 1500 Health Insurance Claim forms.

Once a code is entered here, it will appear on every transaction entry charge. If the default location code is incorrect for the service provided, it may be changed by simply typing in a new location code.

Enter the appropriate code for each of the services you are entering.

Time to Do Procedure—Enter the amount of time it usually takes to perform the procedure. This information is used when scheduling appointments.

Alternate Codes 2/3—If an alternate coding system is used by one or more of the insurance carriers, the alternate codes for the procedure listed can be entered here. The computer can then automatically choose the correct code to enter on the billing form. For example, if the Code Number 2 slot is used for HCPCS codes and the Medicare carrier listed in the Insurance Information file has a 2 in the Procedure Code Type Set, then any HCPCS listed in this spot will automatically print on the billing form for the Medicare carrier.

Taxable—This indicates that the associated item is taxable.

Patient Only Responsible—An X in this box indicates that the patient only is responsible for these charges. Thus, these charges will not be billed to an insurance carrier or show up on a claim form. They will, however, show up on a patient statement or walkout receipt. Examples of charges that may be patient only responsible include cosmetic services, experimental services, dietary services, or charges for a patient missing a scheduled appointment.

Don't Bill to Insurance/Don't Print On—If this procedure should not be charged for certain carriers, you can program the computer to print only for those carriers by inserting an insurance carrier number or a carrier type in this space. Carrier numbers should be separated by commas. For example, if Red is carrier #1, White #2, and Blue #3, and you want this procedure not to print on Red and Blue, then enter 1,3. If this procedure should print only on Medicare, Medicaid, and TRI-CARE/CHAM-PUS billings, enter MAC in this area. When entering Insurance Types, no comma is needed between the letter codes. (For further information on insurance types, see the Insurance Types field under Insurance Carrier List.)

Only Bill to Insurance/Only Print on Insurance—This field works the same as the preceding field, except that this procedure will print only on the carriers listed.

Default Modifiers—If there is a modifier normally associated with this code, enter the modifier here. This will automatically print the modifier on transactions involving this code. If the code is not correct for a given transaction, it may be deleted by simply typing over it.

HIPAA Approved—Checking this box indicates that this code is HIPAA approved.

Revenue Code—Enter the revenue code associated with this procedure. This will be used when billing UB-92 or hospital claims.

Default Units—Enter the common number of units associated with this procedure. This will most often be 1. If the code is not correct for a given transaction, it may be deleted by simply typing over it.

Purchased Service—Enter a check in the box if this procedure is a service purchased from another entity (i.e., a procedure done by an outside lab).

Amounts Screen

Charge Amounts A—Enter the standard charge for the procedure in this field. This charge will automatically show up when the procedure is entered into the Transaction Entry screen. If a different amount is to be charged for an individual customer, this default can always be overridden by simply typing in the new charge. Be aware that CHS has a standard charge for all procedures, but not all doctors in the CHS family will charge the same amount for the same procedures. Doctors set their own prices. Therefore, you should check the amount the provider chooses to bill when entering charges in the Transaction Entry screen. This amount will be listed on the claims next to the description of the service.

Cost of Service/Product—Enter here the practice's cost of providing this service or their cost for a product. This can include the cost of outside lab services or the cost of supplies and other items that are used in conjunction with this service (i.e., cotton swabs, tongue depressors, etc.). This field is optional and is used to help a practice establish how much they are actually making on the services provided.

Medicare Allowed Amount—Enter the amount allowed by Medicare for this procedure if you are a participating provider. If you are not a participating provider, enter the amount that you are allowed to bill Medicare patients for this procedure. This is usually the Medicare allowed amount plus 15%, which you may balance bill the patient. This field helps to calculate any write-off between the standard billed amount and the Medicare-approved amount.

After entering procedure, payment, or adjustment data, be sure to hit **F3** to save, or click on the **Save** button. Your information will then be added to the Procedure/Payment/Adjustment List, which will appear on the screen.

To exit the Procedure/Payment/Adjustment screen, click on the **Close** button.

Exercise 5-6

Using the Procedure/Payment/Adjustment List Screen located under the Lists function on the menu bar, input the procedure codes and accounting codes for the descriptions given in the following list.

Description	Procedure Code	Acctg Code
Patient Check Payment	PT CHECK	1020
Payment By Cash	CASH	1010
Insurance Payment	INS PMT	1030
Standard Adjustment	ADJ STD	1070
Insurance Adjustment	ADJ INS	1080
Check Copayment	COPAY CK	1060
Cash Copayment	COPAY CASH	1090
Inside Lab Charges	LAB IN	1110
Outside Lab Charges	LAB OUT	1100
Comment	COMMENT	NO CODE
Credit Card Payment	CREDIT PMT	1040

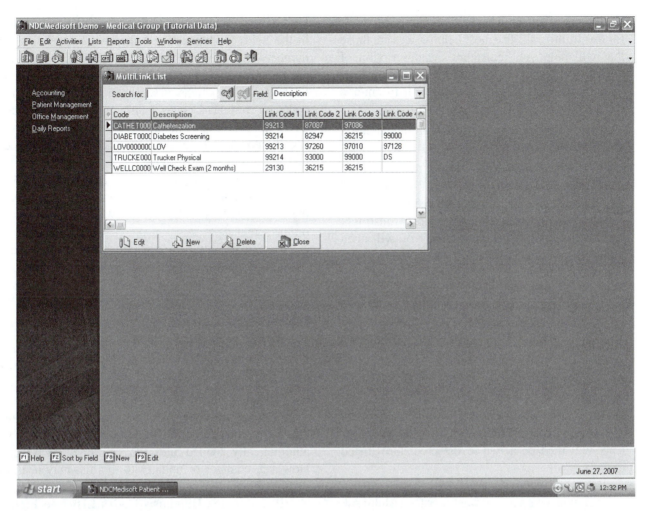

■ **Figure 5–7**   MultiLink List

MultiLink List

When a certain diagnosis is suspected or confirmed, a set of routine procedures are often all performed together. This screen allows the practice to enter a single code for the procedures that, when entered in the Transaction Entry screen, will list all the procedures.

This eliminates having the biller enter each of the procedures one at a time. It also prevents a code from being inadvertently left off the list.

To enter the **MultiLink List (see Figure 5–7),** click the **Lists** menu option and choose **MultiLink Codes**.

Exercise 5–7

Allotta Payne M.D., OB-GYN has asked that the following information be entered into a MultiLink screen. These procedures are always performed together when a patient is pregnant. She has provided a description of the procedures, but is unsure of the proper CPT® codes for them. Look up the proper CPT® codes and then enter the data into the MultiLink Screen.

Description	CPT® Code
Office Visit, mod complexity	_____
Urinalysis	_____
Obstetric Lab Panel	_____

Code—Enter an alphabetical or numerical code for this MultiLink. The most helpful ones are those that will help you remember the description of what the MultiLink is for (i.e., DIABSCR for Diabetes Screening). If you do not wish to enter a code, the computer will assign one for you.

Description—Enter a description of the diagnosis or condition.

Link Code 1/2/3/4/5/6/7—Enter the procedure codes associated with this MultiLink. Each of the procedure codes must have been previously entered into the Procedure/Payment/Adjustment Codes List. If they have not been, you will need to add them before entering the codes here. If the codes have been entered but you are unsure of the code, use **F6** or the magnifying glass icon to search for the procedure. To add a new code to the Procedure/Payment/Adjustment Codes List without backing out of this screen, use the **F8** key.

Link Code #8—Enter the eighth code associated with this MultiLink. If more than eight codes are needed, enter the MultiLink code for an additional MultiLink. All procedures in this secondary MultiLink will then be added to the procedures listed earlier.

For example, let's say you want to enter a MultiLink for the procedures performed for an unexplained death, and there are 10 separate procedures done (requiring 10 separate codes). You would name the MultiLink code UNEXDTH. Then enter the first seven procedure codes in the fields for link codes 1 through 7. On link code number 8, you would enter UNEXDTH2. You then create a second MultiLink entry under the code UNEXDTH2 in which you will enter the remaining three codes on MultiLink codes 1 through 3. When the code UNEXDTH is entered into the Transaction Entry screen, it will automatically print all 10 codes on separate lines on the Transaction Entry screen.

After entering MultiLink data, be sure to hit **F3** to save, or click on the **Save** button. Your information will then be added to the MultiLink List, which will appear on the screen.

To exit the MultiLink screen, click on the **Close** button at the bottom of the screen.

Diagnosis List

This list contains the ICD-9-CM codes that represent a diagnosis of the illness or condition the patient is being treated for. This screen allows you to enter data on each diagnosis used in treating patients. In the real world, many providers and medical billers will purchase computerized ICD-9-CM code lists that can be automatically loaded into the computer each year. However, changes or updates to this list may need to be done manually.

To access the **Diagnosis Codes List (see Figure 5–8)**, click on the Diagnosis Codes List icon, or choose the **Lists** menu option and choose **Diagnosis Codes**.

Exercise 5-8

Sue Pervisor gives you a list of diagnoses that were not entered into the system (Document 4). Look up the correct ICD-9-CM codes and enter the information for these diagnoses in the appropriate fields in the Diagnosis Codes List.

Code 1—Enter the diagnosis code, including any periods or additional classification numbers.

Description—Enter a description of the diagnosis. You are given more room than appears in the field. If you continue typing after hitting the field margin, the items first entered will scroll off the left side of the field, but will still be included in the complete description. However, it is important to be sure that all the pertinent data is included in the first part of the description line. When using the search feature, the first set of characters is the only one to appear on the screen. Additionally, on many billing forms and reports, only the first part of the diagnosis appears. The remaining information will only appear on a walkout receipt that is printed in paragraph form.

Alternate Codes Sets: Code 2/3—If an alternate coding system is used by one or more of the insurance carriers, the alternate codes for the procedure listed can be entered here. The computer can then automatically choose the correct code to enter on the billing form. For example, if the Code Number 2 slot is used for state-assigned codes and the insurance carrier listed in the Insurance Information file has a 2 in the Procedure Code Type Set, then any state-assigned codes listed in this spot will automatically print on the billing form for that insurance carrier.

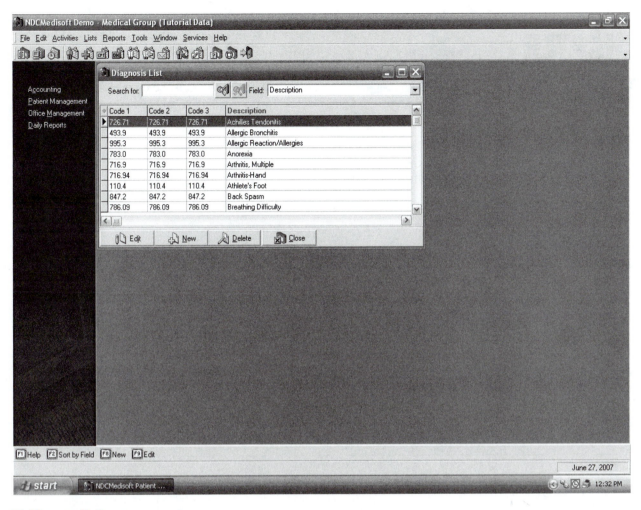

■ **Figure 5–8**   Diagnosis List

HIPAA Approved—Checking this box indicates that this code is HIPAA approved.

Inactive Code—Check this box if you need to deactivate a code, but not delete it. This may need to be done if an ICD-9-CM code has been deleted by the World Health Organization (WHO), but all previous claims with this code have not yet been paid. If there are still open issues on the claims, the code needs to remain in the system. Having a code on an inactive status may prevent you from entering this code on new claims.

After entering diagnosis data, be sure to hit **F3** to save, or click on the **Save** button. Your information will then be added to the Diagnosis Code List, which will appear on the screen.

To exit the Diagnosis Code screen, click on the **Close** button.

CHAPTER REVIEW

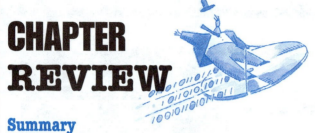

ers, addresses, procedure codes, and diagnoses. The information entered in these screens will be used to bill for the procedures performed by a provider and to keep track of patient accounts. Data usually must be entered in these screens prior to being accessed in the Transaction Entry and Billing screens.

Summary

- The Lists menu choices allow you to enter information on the patient, providers, insurance carri-

Questions for Review

Directions: Answer the following questions without looking back into the material just covered. Write your answers in the space provided.

1. What does EDI/EMC stand for?

_____

_____

_____

_____

2. In the Address List, what is a facility?

_____

_____

_____

_____

3. Name five advantages of EDI/EMC claims over paper claims.

1. _____

_____

_____

_____

2. _____

_____

_____

_____

3. _____

_____

_____

_____

4. _____

_____

_____

_____

5. _____

_____

_____

_____

4. What is the function of a clearinghouse?

_____

_____

_____

_____

_____

5. What types of services would be considered patient only responsibility?

_____

_____

_____

_____

_____

If you were unable to answer any of the questions, refer back to that section, and then fill in the answers.

6
Patients/Guarantors and Cases List

After completion of this chapter
you will be able to:

- Enter information on patients, guarantors, and cases.
- Demonstrate use of the patient recall list.

Each patient and guarantor must be set up in this list to be accessed. The Patient List has two screens, containing all the data necessary to keep an accurate and complete patient file. Because the Patient Information and Case screens are so important, they will each be handled in their own chapter. The remaining Lists Screens were covered in Chapter 5.

Case-Based Files

MediSoft for Windows allows for patient files to be set up on a case basis. This means that you can track information regarding treatment on a specific incident. You can also keep track of two incidents and bill two separate insurance carriers.

For example, a patient may be seen on a regular basis for a diagnosis of hypertension. Then suddenly he has an injury at work. Although his regular insurance carrier would be responsible for payment on all treatments relating to the hypertension, the employer's compensation carrier would be responsible for payment on the services relating to the treatment of the work injury.

By setting up two separate case files for this patient, it is easy to keep the hypertension charges separate from the compensation charges.

Depending on the circumstances of patient visits, a patient may have any number of files. Some practices choose to combine all patient visits under one file, unless they are billing a different insurance carrier.

Although the case-based file scenario allows for easy tracking of individual diagnoses and/or conditions, it can make it more confusing to track the number of times a patient visits the provider. Therefore, the provider should consider carefully when they want to establish a new case. For purposes of this text, all patients should be given a separate case file for each of the following situations:

1. Routine office visits and/or short-term conditions/diseases (i.e., flu) should be lumped together under a single case file.

2. Chronic or long-term conditions or diagnoses (those lasting longer than six months, such as pregnancy, diabetes, etc.) should each have their own separate case file.

3. Workers' compensation cases (including those that may possibly be related to compensation) should be placed in a separate case file.

4. Accidents, especially those in which a third party may be at fault, should be placed in a separate case file.

Because the simulated work program encompasses such a short period of time, most patients will only have a single case file. However, care should be taken to remember the four situations listed earlier, as some of them will be used, and thus separate case files will need to be set up for certain patients.

Patients/Guarantors and Cases List

The **Patients/Guarantors and Cases List (see Figure 6–1)** allows you to enter data on a patient. It contains all the personal information needed on the patient, as well as additional information regarding specific encounters. Each patient and each guarantor, whether they are a patient or not, must have their information set up in a file.

This menu option actually contains two separate lists, which have their own data fields. The first is for entering information on patients and guarantors. The second is for entering more specific information regarding a case, the insurance carriers responsible for payment on the case, and other information.

Searching for a patient and deleting a patient are performed here in a similar manner to all other lists. (For further information, refer to Chapter 5.) However, once a patient is chosen in the search field, a list of that patient's cases will appear in a second search screen to the right of the patient's name. This allows you to choose not only the patient you wish to work on, but also the specific case.

If you wish to add a new patient, simply click on **New** or press **F8** while the cursor is in the patient portion of the screen. If you wish to add a new case to an existing patient, highlight the patient's name in the Case portion of the screen. The options at the bottom of the screen will now change to Edit Case, New Case, Delete Case, or Copy Case. This allows you to perform these functions without changing the patient information.

Patient/Guarantor List

There are two screens in the Patient/Guarantor List: the Name, Address screen and the Other Information screen.

Exercise 6-1

Take out the patient information sheet for the Dunnitt family (Document 5). As you go through each of the following fields, enter the patient information as it pertains to the family. Each of the family members must be entered separately under their own patient chart number. Read through the description detailing each screen, whether it pertains to this patient or not. It will help to familiarize you with the MediSoft system and its capabilities.

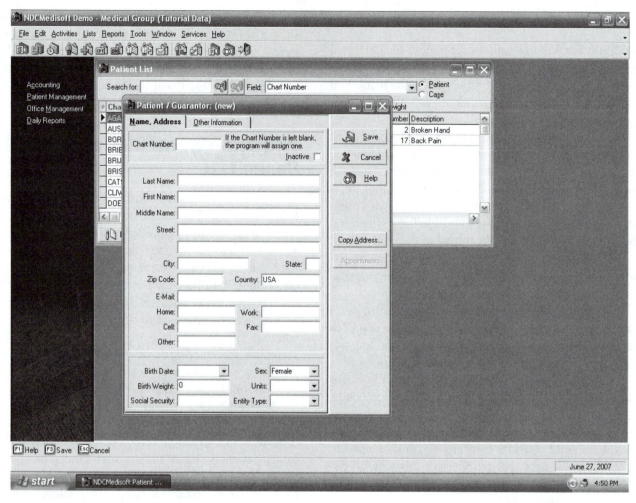

■ **Figure 6-1** Patient/Guarantor

Not all screens or fields will be affected by the information given. For example, if the patient is not currently being treated, the condition screen may not be utilized. Also, there may not be any secondary or tertiary insurance coverage for family members.

Name, Address Screen

This screen is used for entering the patient's name and address, as well as other personal information about the patient.

Chart Number: Patients must have their own individual patient chart number. Due to the configuration of the MediSoft system, each patient chart number must have eight digits (either letters or numbers). Each provider may choose their own system for setting up patient accounts, or you can allow MediSoft to assign chart numbers for each patient. For this course we will allow MediSoft to assign patient chart numbers. Be sure to write the patient chart number on the Patient Information Sheet.

Inactive: Check this box if you need to deactivate a patient, but not delete him/her. This may need to be done if a patient is no longer with the practice, but all the claims have not yet been paid. If there are still open issues on the claims of this patient, the patient needs to remain in the system. Having a patient on an inactive status may prevent you from entering new claims for this patient.

Last Name: Enter the last name of the patient. If the patient has a title designation at the end of their name (i.e., M.D., Jr., Sr., etc.), it should be entered directly after the last name.

First Name: Enter the patient's first name.

Middle Initial: Enter the patient's middle initial.

Street: Enter the street address of the patient.

City: Enter the city the patient lives in.

State: Enter the state in which the patient lives. This should coincide with the official postal two-letter state abbreviation.

Zip Code: Enter the patient's zip code. If the complete nine-digit zip code is known, enter the first five digits, a hyphen, and the remaining four digits.

Country: Enter the country in which the patient resides. This information is optional, but could be helpful for providers whose practices are near a country border.

E-mail: Enter the patient's e-mail address.

Home: Enter the patient's home phone number. Do not use parentheses or hyphens.

Work: If there is a work/office phone number for the patient, enter it here. Do not use parentheses or hyphens.

Cell: Enter the patient's personal cell phone number. Do not use parentheses or hyphens.

Fax: Enter the patient's fax phone number. Do not use parentheses or hyphens.

Other: Enter any other contact numbers for this patient (i.e., a pager number). Do not use parentheses or hyphens.

Birth Date: Enter the patient's birth date in the MMDDCCYY format. If desired, you may click on the calendar to bring up and choose a date in the same manner you chose the date under File/Set Program Date.

Sex: Enter the sex of the patient: M for male, F for female. This should be the gender of the patient at the time services were rendered. If a patient enters the hospital for a sex change operation, it should be the gender of the patient as of the date they entered the hospital.

Birth Weight: Enter the birth weight of the patient, if known. This field is used for newborns or infants.

Units: Choose either grams or pounds to indicate the correct units for the weight entered in the previous field.

Social Security Number: Enter the patient's Social Security number. Do not enter hyphens.

Other Information Screen

This screen is used to indicate assigned provider, signature on file, and employment information on the patient or guarantor.

Type: Choose whether this person is a patient or a guarantor. A guarantor is someone who is financially responsible for a patient (i.e., a parent or guardian). This box is important when a dependent is being treated. However, information for the insured is needed to properly process the insurance claims.

1. What other instances can you think of where the patient may not be the guarantor?

_____

_____

_____

_____

Assigned Provider: Enter the code (from the provider listing) that corresponds to the doctor who is assigned to this patient. This information will automatically be transferred to the transaction entry and onto the billing forms. If another provider within the practice sees a patient (i.e., a patient is referred to a specialist within the group), this information will need to be changed so that the proper provider shows up on the patient's billing.

Patient ID #2: This box is an optional method for searching for a patient. Instead of searching for a patient by the chart number or the patient name, any key or combination of keys can be entered into this box to search for the patient. This can be a complete last name, nickname, company affiliation, or any other way that makes it easier to locate the record. This box is for internal use only and does not show up on insurance billing forms.

Patient Billing Code: This field allows you to sort patients into separate fields. The actual choice of groups was made in the Billing Codes field of the Lists Menu option. This field allows you to assign a patient to a specific group.

Patient Indicator: This field can be used as an additional sorting tool. You can create a five-digit code for any type of group.

For example: If you enter MEDCR and the Billing Code for this patient was Last Name A–M, sorting by both of these fields would allow you to locate all the Medicare patients whose last names began with A–M.

Healthcare ID: This is a code to help you identify the patient without revealing information about their identity (which may not be the case with a patient account number). This field has been created to help a practice maintain HIPAA compliance.

Signature on File: Place an X in the box if the patient's signature is on file authorizing release of medical information. If the patient's signature is not on file, the patient must sign the form prior to submitting it to the insurance carrier.

Signature Date: Enter the date on which the patient or guarantor signed the Release of Medical Information form. The signature on these forms is generally good for a period of one year unless stated otherwise on the form. A patient may revoke this signature by writing a letter to the practice stating that they no longer authorize the release of their information. This box is only activated if an X is placed in the Signature on File box.

Emergency Contact

The following fields allow you to enter emergency contact information for the patient.

Name: Enter the full name of the patient's emergency contact.

Home Phone: Enter the home phone number of the patient's emergency contact. Do not use parentheses or hyphens.

Cell Phone: Enter the cell phone number of the patient's emergency contact. Do not use parentheses or hyphens.

Default Employment Information for New Cases

Employer: Enter the employer address code. This item cross-references with information entered in the Addresses List. If this information has not yet been entered, you should enter it before you proceed.

You can press **F6** to search for an employer address code or click on the magnifying glass to the right of this field. If the correct employer has not been entered, press **F8**, and the Address List screen will appear. This will allow you to enter the new address before going on. (For instructions on completing the Address List screen, see Address List.)

Status: Most group insurance issued through an employer requires that the insured work full time

for the company. Additionally, dependents who work full time may have duplicate coverage with their employer. Use this box to show the patient's work status as follows:

- Not Employed
- Full-time
- Part-time
- Retired
- Unknown

Work Phone: Indicate the work phone number for the patient. Do not use parentheses or hyphens.

Extension: Indicate the extension number at which the patient can be reached at work.

Location: This field can be used to indicate where in a company a person works. This can be an actual site (i.e., Tucson to indicate the patient works in the Tucson office), or a location within a site (i.e., warehouse, shop, or the name of a department).

Retirement Date: If the retirement date is known for this patient, indicate it here. This allows you to know when their insurance may terminate or may change to a different plan. If a patient retires or terminates, but elects to continue coverage under the Consolidated Omnibus Budget Reconciliation Act (COBRA) rules, the biller should contact the employer to ensure that the current monthly premium has been paid prior to the rendering of services. COBRA coverage can last for up to 18, 29, or 36 months, depending on the circumstances.

Case Screens

Once you have entered the basic data on the patient, you need to enter the information regarding this case of treatment. If this person is the guarantor and not the patient, you will not need to access these screens.

The case screens will need to be completed to provide all the necessary information for completing the 1500 Health Insurance Claim form. Because some items on the form pertain to individual situations, having separate case screens allows you to keep each item separate.

Although it may not be wise to create a new case file for each separate diagnosis of a patient, certain situations will necessitate the creation of a separate case file. These can include the following:

1. **Standard Treatment.** All standard treatment for a patient should be kept under one case. Even if the specific incidents or reasons for treatment are not

related, keeping items together can allow you to see the overall health of a patient and their treatment history.

2. **Chronic Condition.** If a patient is receiving treatment for an ongoing (chronic) condition (i.e., diabetes), the provider may want this information entered into a separate case file. All treatments relating to this specific diagnosis can then be tracked. This may include regular checkups or eventual blindness or amputation of a limb.

3. **Motor Vehicle Accident.** Often there is a third-party liability or other insurance (i.e., auto insurance) that may cover some or all of the costs related to a motor vehicle accident. Therefore, all treatment for injuries received in a specific motor vehicle accident should be kept separate from all other treatments.

4. **Workers' Compensation/Work-Related Injury.** Any injury received on the job or that is related to

work is often covered by the employer's compensation policy. Treatment for these injuries should be separated from all other treatment so that the employer's insurance carrier can be accurately billed.

Personal Screen

This screen allows you to enter personal data regarding the patient and this specific case (**see Figure 6–2**).

Case Number: The MediSoft program will automatically assign a case number. These numbers begin with one and continue consecutively.

Description: Enter a brief description of this case. This will help you to locate the proper case when using the search screen.

Guarantor: Enter the chart number for the guarantor for this treatment episode. For a guarantor chart number to work, the guarantor must have

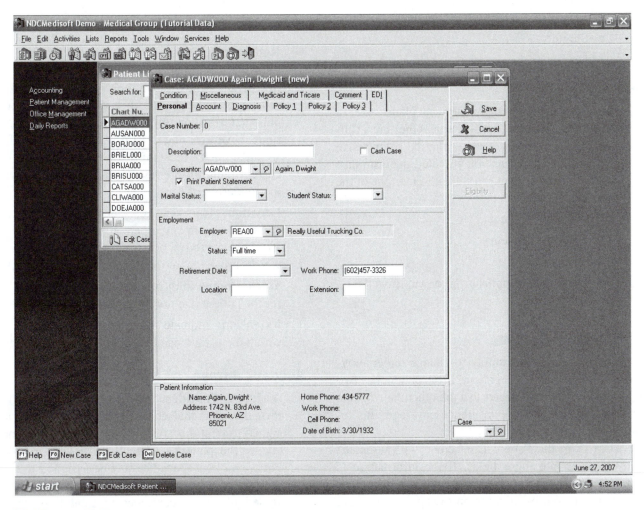

■ **Figure 6–2**   Personal Case Screen

been previously entered as a patient or a guarantor in the Patient List. MediSoft will automatically enter the chart number of the patient. If this is incorrect, simply change it by typing in a new chart number or by searching for the correct chart number. You can easily access the search feature by clicking on the magnifying glass to the right of this field.

Print Patient Statement: If a patient or family should not receive a monthly statement, leave this box blank. If they should receive a statement, place an X in the box. This is an on/off field. Each time you click on the field, the X will appear or disappear. All CHS patients should receive statements.

Marital Status: Enter the marital status designation for the patient. These marital status designations correspond with those accepted on the 1500 Health Insurance Claim form as follows:

- Divorced
- Legally Separated
- Married
- Single
- Unknown
- Widowed

Student Status: Many insurance plans cover a dependent until age 18 or 19, unless they are a full-time student. Then coverage may be extended to age 23 or 24. This question will alert the insurance carrier that the patient is a student. Enter one of the following:

- Full-time Student
- Part-time Student
- Nonstudent
- If the student status is unknown, leave the field blank

Employment Section

Here you have an opportunity to change the employment information for the patient. If the patient has two jobs and this accident relates to a job other than the one through which they have insurance coverage, this information could be important.

Data from the Patient List screen will automatically transfer into these fields. If the information is correct, simply tab past these fields. If it is incorrect, you can change it by clicking on the appropriate field and reentering the data.

Employer: Enter the employer address code. This item cross-references with information entered in the Addresses List. If this information has not yet been entered, you should enter it before you proceed.

You can press **F6** to search for an employer address or click on the magnifying glass to the right of this field. If the correct employer has not been entered, press **F8**, and the Address List screen will appear. This will allow you to enter the new address before going on.

Status: Most group insurance issued through an employer requires that the insured work full time for the company. Additionally, dependents who work full time may have duplicate coverage with their employer. Use this box to show the patient's work status as follows:

- Not Employed
- Full-time
- Part-time
- Retired
- Unknown

Retirement Date: If the retirement date is known for this patient, indicate it here. This allows you to know when their insurance may terminate or may change to a different plan. If a patient retires or terminates, but elects to continue coverage under COBRA rules, the biller should contact the employer to ensure that the current monthly premium has been paid prior to the rendering of services.

Location: This field can be used to indicate where in a company a person works. This can be an actual site (city), or a location within a site (i.e., warehouse, shop, or the name of a department).

Work Phone: Indicate the work phone number for the patient. Do not use parentheses or hyphens.

Extension: Indicate the extension number at which the patient can be reached at work.

Account Screen

Assigned Provider: Enter the code (from the Provider List) that corresponds to the doctor assigned to treat this specific case. This may or may not be the patient's normally assigned provider. For example, a specialist may be assigned to treat the patient's heart disease, but his regularly assigned physician continues to treat him for all other conditions (**see Figure 6–3**).

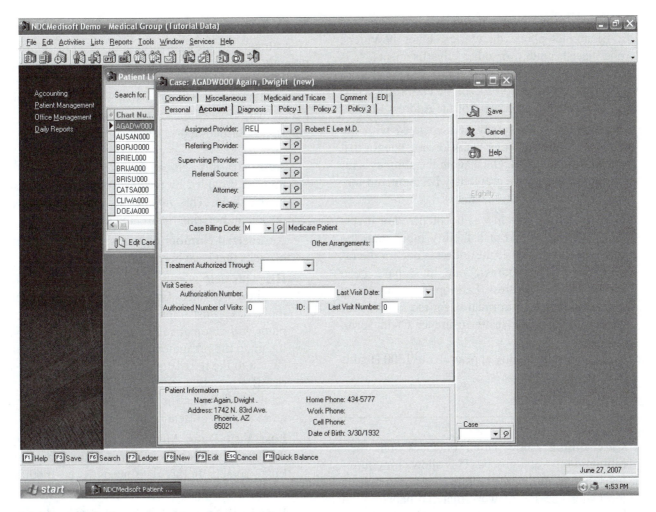

■ Figure 6–3   Account Screen

If the provider has not been previously added to the Provider List, they will need to be added using the **F8** key.

Once the provider's code has been entered, the provider's name will appear to the right of the code.

Referring Provider: If this patient was referred by another provider, the referring physician and their UPIN need to be indicated on the billing forms (especially on Medicare claims). To use this field, the referring physician's information must have previously been entered in the Referring Providers List. If so, enter the physician's Referring Provider Code into this field.

If the referring provider has not been entered into the Referring Provider list, they will need to be added using the **F8** key.

2. Where does this information appear on a 1500 Health Insurance Claim form?

Supervising Provider: At times the work will be performed by one provider under the direction of another provider (i.e., a practitioner's assistant may provide services under the direction of the physician). In such a case, the supervising provider's code will be entered here. This provider's information must have previously been entered into the provider listing.

Referral Source: Enter the Address Code for the person or entity that referred this patient. To have an Address Code, the person or entity must have been previously entered using the Address Lists screen. If they have not been entered, you can enter them by pressing the **F8** key.

This field is used to track how effective your advertising sources are. To gain the most effective report, entries must be identical. For example, if the patient was referred by a Yellow Pages ad, all patients with the referral "Yellow Pages" will appear in a different listing from those referred by

"Phone Listing." Common referral sources include a friend, telephone directories, other providers, pharmacists, radio, or other advertisements. It is possible to create a referral source for the preceding by placing the words "Yellow Pages" (or whatever else) in the name field of the Address List.

Attorney: If an attorney is associated with the care of this patient, enter the Address Code for that attorney in this field. Once again the attorney's information must have previously been entered into the Address Information database.

Facility: If the patient was hospitalized or if services were provided at a facility other than the provider's office, enter the address code for the facility here. The address code must have been created in the Address List option. The entire name and address information for the facility will appear on the 1500 Health Insurance Claim form.

3. Where does the facility appear on the 1500 Health Insurance Claim form?

Case Billing Code: Often practices split their billing into several groups. This allows for continuous income during the month, as well as prevents the major backlog of work that can happen with billing all patients at once. Using this field, you can place patients into groups for billing purposes. Patients can be grouped together by last name (i.e., A–M is billed on the first of the month, and N–Z is billed on the 15th of the month), insurance carrier or type of insurance, or any other form the practice wishes. The billing code must have been previously entered in the Billing Code List. Because we are using so few patients, we will bill them all at once. Therefore, you may leave this space blank.

Other Arrangements: Four characters are allowed in this field to indicate any special arrangements that have been made with the patient. These can involve items such as discounts, payment programs, or courtesy services (no billing). When new charges are entered for the patient on the Transaction Entry screen, this code is displayed at the bottom of the screen to remind you of the arrangements that have been made.

Treatment Authorized Through: Enter the date through which the insurance carrier has authorized treatments. Treatments received after this date may not be paid by the insurance carrier.

Visit Series

If treatment for the patient requires a series of visits, preauthorization may be needed to determine the number of treatments the insurance carrier will cover (i.e., up to 12 massage therapy visits may be covered for a patient with a back injury). The following fields are for entering information on a series of visits.

Authorization Number: The preauthorization number provided by the carrier should be entered in this field. This number usually identifies the person authorizing the treatments.

Authorized Number of Visits: Enter the number of visits that have been authorized.

ID: This field allows for several visit series to be monitored at once. Enter a letter A–Z to indicate the series. Most often an A is entered. The computer will automatically count the number of visits, up to the preauthorized limit number, and then switch to the next letter in the series. Different series IDs may be used for subsequent series of the same problem or for different problems that require a series of treatments.

Last Visit Date: MediSoft automatically enters the date of the last visit entered in the Transaction Entry screen. If this date needs to be modified, enter the corrected information.

Last Visit Number: Each time a visit is entered in the Transaction Entry screen, this number is increased by one until it reaches the limit entered in the Authorized Number of Visits field. This number is normally not edited by the medical biller.

Diagnosis Screen

This screen is for entering diagnoses and codes associated with this patient's treatment (see **Figure 6–4**).

Default Diagnosis 1, 2, 3, and 4: These fields are for entering the patient's diagnoses. Because MediSoft handles charges on a case basis, often the diagnoses for all treatments within a case will be the same. Because many cases will relate to the same diagnoses, entering the diagnoses in this field will save time. Enter the diagnosis codes associated with this patient. If no code is entered, the diagnosis entered during the first transaction entry will automatically become the default code and will be entered in the first space.

Be sure to check default diagnosis codes with each new visit, as ICD-9-CM codes can change each year.

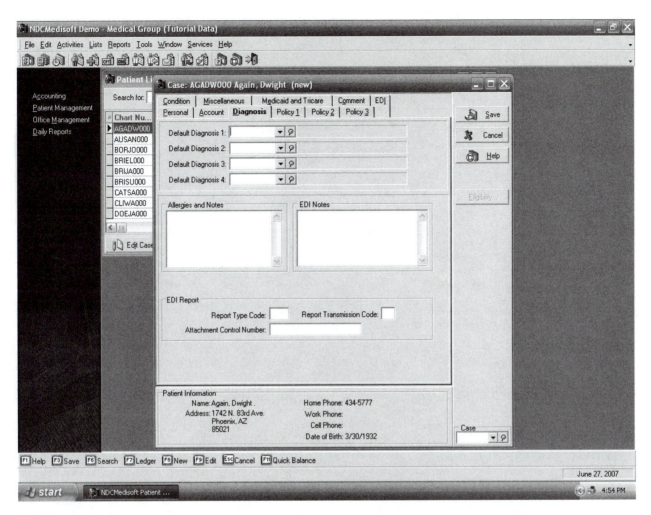

■ **Figure 6–4**   Diagnosis Screen

Allergies and Notes: Enter any allergies or special notes associated with this patient. This information will appear at the bottom of the Transaction Entry screen, but it will not print anywhere. While entering the information for the Dunnitt and Waite families, be sure to check whether any data should be entered here.

EDI/EMC Notes

This window allows the entry of additional data that is included with electronic claims when they are submitted. If the provider is an anesthesiologist, enter the symbol @ (shift 2). The first 17 characters entered after this symbol will print on the claim form. This allows entry of documentation such as Time: 12:00–14:50, which is needed for claim processing.

If the practice type in the Practice Information screen was listed as Chiropractic, an additional field will be added for **Level of Subluxation**. A subluxation is a partial or incomplete dislocation; although this can

occur anywhere in the body, chiropractors treat subluxations of the spine. The subluxation level is indicated by where the subluxation occurs (C1, T2, L3, etc.). This information is often required by insurance carriers when a patient is treated by a chiropractor.

Using a medical dictionary and/or other resource materials, answer the following questions.

4. What does subluxation mean?

_____

_____

5. What do the terms C1, T2, and L3 mean, and where in the body are they located?

_____

_____

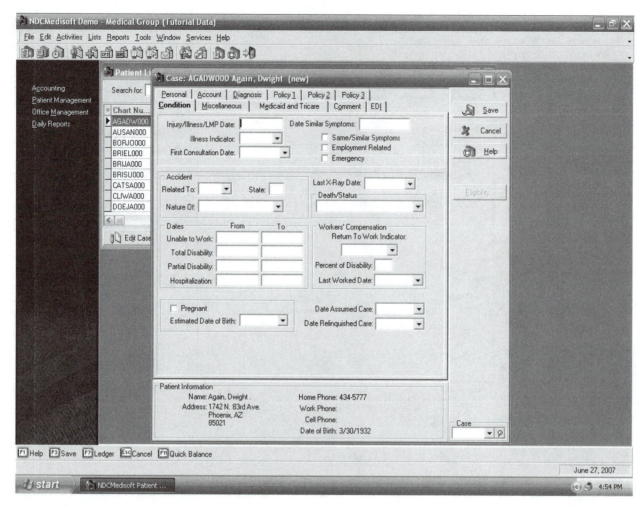

■ **Figure 6–5** Condition Screen

Condition Screen

This screen contains information that pertains to this specific episode of treatment (**see Figure 6–5**). This information is used to properly complete the 1500 Health Insurance Claim form. At this time, you will not enter condition information for the Dunnitt and Waite families. This data will be completed when treatment commences.

While reading through this section, compare these fields with the boxes to be completed on the 1500 Health Insurance Claim form. Next to each item, indicate the 1500 Health Insurance Claim form box number. If there is no corresponding box number on the

1500 Health Insurance Claim form, enter NONE on the line given.

Injury/Illness/LMP Date: Enter the date on which the illness or injury occurred. If this condition is related to a pregnancy, enter the date of the patient's last menstrual period (LMP). If the onset of the illness was gradual, enter a G, and the word *gradual* will appear on the form. Entering N will print N/A in this field.

6. Where does this information appear on a 1500 Health Insurance Claim form?

_____

Illness Indicator: Enter an *I* to indicate if the date given in the previous box pertains to an illness or injury. Enter an *L* to indicate the date is the last menstrual period, or you may click on the *p* to the right of the field, and a list of these choices will appear.

First Consultation Date: Enter the date on which the provider first began treating this patient for this condition.

Date Similar Symptoms: If the patient has had similar symptoms in the past that are not related to this specific episode of treatment (i.e., tonsillitis patient had a previous tonsillitis experience two years ago), enter the date those symptoms occurred.

7. Where does this information appear on a 1500 Health Insurance Claim form?

_____

Same/Similar Symptoms: Enter an *X* in this box for Yes; similar symptoms occurred on the date entered. Leave the box blank if no similar symptoms have appeared.

Employment Related: Enter an *X* in this box if this condition is related to the patient's employment. This is most often used when a person is injured on the job, but the condition could also be a chronic condition that is due to their job. For example, if a person repeatedly uses their fingers to type, they may suddenly be seized with a sharp pain in their wrist while doing weekend gardening. The doctor may diagnose the condition as carpal tunnel syndrome. Although the initial reason for visiting the doctor was pain from gardening, the underlying cause of the condition is likely the constant typing done while at work.

If the condition is work related, workers' compensation laws may cover payment on this claim. An empty box indicates the claim is not work related.

8. Where does this information appear on a 1500 Health Insurance Claim form?

_____

Emergency: Enter an *X* in this box if these procedures were provided on an emergency basis. Leave the box blank if they were not.

9. Where does this information appear on a 1500 Health Insurance Claim form?

_____

Accident Information

If these services were related to an accident, information regarding the accident can be entered in this section.

Related To: Enter a *Y* if this claim is related to an accident, an *A* if it is related to an auto accident, and an *N* if it is not related to an accident. Or you can click on the ↓ to the right of the field for a list of these choices. It is important to determine the accident status of each and every claim because additional benefits may be available for accidents. Additionally, if the accident involved another party (i.e., an auto accident or negligence on the part of another person or company) third-party liability laws might cover payment on this claim.

10. If an *A* is placed in this box, where will this information appear on a 1500 Health Insurance Claim form?

_____

11. Look at Document 12 in the back of this book. Does the Ball Insurance Carriers contract have an accident benefit? If so, what does it say?

_____

_____

_____

_____

12. How can this benefit affect payment on an accident claim?

_____

_____

_____

_____

State: List the two-digit postal code for the state in which the accident occurred if the accident is auto related. This helps to determine the laws and rules that govern coverage of a two-party accident because many states have different laws and rules.

13. Where does this information appear on a 1500 Health Insurance Claim form?

_____

Nature of Accident: If this claim pertains to an accident, choose one of the following codes:

- Injured at Home
- Injured at School
- Injured during Recreation
- Motorcycle Injury
- Work Injury/Noncollision
- Work Injury/Self-Employed
- Some states require this code when submitting claims electronically

Dates Unable to Work: Enter the beginning and ending dates of the time the patient is unable to work.

14. Where does this information appear on a 1500 Health Insurance Claim form?

_____

Total Disability: Enter the beginning and ending dates of the time the patient is to be considered totally disabled.

Partial Disability: Enter the beginning and ending dates of the time the patient is to be considered partially disabled.

Hospitalization: Enter the admit and discharge dates for a hospitalized patient.

15. Where does this information appear on a 1500 Health Insurance Claim form?

_____

Last X-ray Date: Some insurance carriers require the date of the last x-ray. This is usually for chiropractic patients who are eligible for Medicare. If needed, enter the date of the last x-ray.

Death/Status: D. A. Karnofsky, a twentieth-century physician, developed a scale to indicate a patient's physical state, performance, and prognosis. The scale ranges from 100, perfectly well, to 0, dead. Some carriers require the reporting of the patient's condition on a similar scale. The code to be entered in this box is based on the scale Karnofsky

developed. Appropriate codes are (from worst to best) as follows:

- Dead (Medicare Assigned claims only)
- Moribund (dying)
- Very sick
- Severely disabled
- Disabled
- Requires considerable assistance
- Requires occasional assistance
- Cares for self
- Normal activity with effort
- Able to carry on normal activity
- Normal

Return to Work Indicator: Enter an _L_ if the patient is allowed to return to work with limited activity. Enter an _N_ if the patient is allowed to resume normal work activity. Enter a _C_ if the return to work is conditional. Or you may click on the ↓ to the right of the field to get a list of these choices.

Percent of Disability: Once a patient's condition is stabilized and no additional progress is expected to be made, the physician will list the patient as permanently disabled. This percentage indicator reflects the amount of disability that the patient will likely have for the remainder of their life. This can range from 1 to 2% for a permanently disabled toe to 100% for a totally disabled patient.

Pregnant: Place an X in this box if the patient is pregnant.

Estimated Date of Birth: Enter the estimated date of birth for this pregnancy.

Date Assumed Care/Date Relinquished Care: These fields are provided for situations in which two different providers share the care of one episode of treatment. For example, one provider is responsible for the antepartum care and delivery, and a different provider is responsible for the postpartum care. These fields allow you to indicate the dates a specific provider assumed and relinquished care for the patient.

Miscellaneous Screen

This screen is used for additional information relating to this claim or this case of treatment (see **Figure 6–6**).

Outside Lab Work: Enter an X in this box if an outside lab billed for services related to this claim.

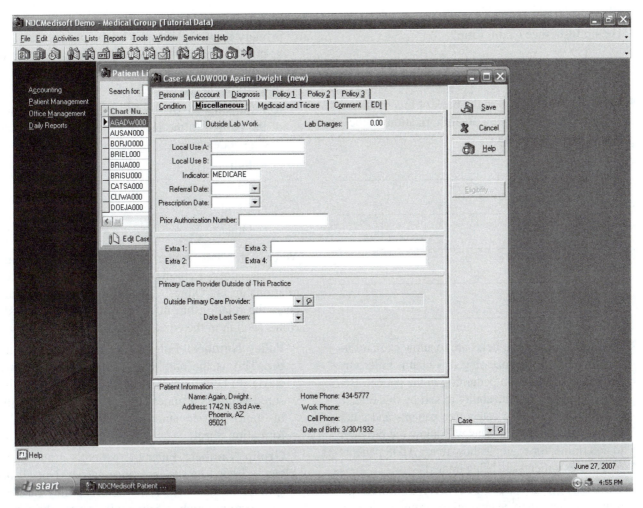

■ **Figure 6–6**   Miscellaneous Screen

16. Where does this information appear on a 1500 Health Insurance Claim form?

_____

Lab Charges: Enter the amount of the outside lab charges in this box.

17. Where does this information appear on a 1500 Health Insurance Claim form?

_____

Local Use A: This box completes any information needed for item 10d on the 1500 Health Insurance Claim Form. Currently this box is used by Medicare to indicate secondary payers or items needed to process Medicare claims. If this item is required by your Medicare carrier, they will specify the code or item they want in this field.

Local Use B: This box completes any information needed for item 19 on the 1500 Health Insurance Claim form. This box is used by states and localities to indicate information they need in claim processing.

Indicator: If further delineation is needed in setting up billing cycles, this field may be used with the Billing Code field to create an unlimited array of billing groups.

Referral Date: Enter the date of referral.

Prescription Date: Enter the date a prescription was given.

Prior Authorization #: If preauthorization is required for certain procedures or treatments, a preauthorization number will be supplied by the carrier in regard to these services. If a preauthorization number has been obtained for any of the services on this claim, enter the number in this box. Preauthorization is also sometimes called precertification.

18. Where does this information appear on a 1500 Health Insurance Claim form?

_____

19. Look at Document 13 in the back of this book. What procedures require preauthorization on the Rover Insurers contract?

_____

_____

_____

_____

Extra 1/2/3/4: These fields are to allow extra information needed in processing this claim. Enter any additional information pertaining to the patient. Because MediSoft has the ability to sort by this field, a provider may wish to categorize patients and enter certain categories here. This will allow the provider to determine, for example, how many AIDS patients or diabetes patients are being treated.

Outside Primary Care Provider: This field allows information to be entered regarding a primary care provider for the patient who is not a member of this practice. This field is most often used when the provider is a specialist and was referred by an outside primary care physician. This space is for the address code. To enter this provider, their information must have previously been entered in the Address List screen.

Date Last Seen: Enter the date this patient was last seen by the outside primary care provider.

Policy 1 Screen (H2)

This screen allows you to enter information on the primary insurance coverage for this patient (**see Figure 6–7**).

Insurance 1: Enter the code number for the insurance company. The code number comes from the Insurance Carriers List. If you are unsure of the insurance carrier number, press **F6** or click on the magnifying glass and search for it. If the insurance carrier has not been entered, press **F8** to add the insurance carrier.

Policy Holder 1: Enter the chart number of the primary insured. This may be the patient (self), or a spouse or parent of the patient. Enter the correct patient chart number, or press **F6** (or click on the magnifying glass) to search for it.

Relationship to Insured: Enter the relationship of the patient to the insured according to the following code choices:

- Self
- Spouse
- Child
- Other

Note: In this case, the term "Child" includes natural children, adopted children, and stepchildren. If the relationship is "Other," it would be appropriate to enter the relationship information in the Allergies/Notes section in the condition screen.

Policy Number: Enter the patient's policy number. This is the number issued by the insurance carrier to help them keep track of the plan the insured is covered under. This is the ID# under the insurance carrier name located on the Patient Information Sheet.

Group Number: Enter the patient's group number as issued by the insurance carrier. Not all insurance carriers will issue both a policy number and a group number. Some will issue only one or the other, and some will issue a group name rather than a group number.

Claim Number: This field is required for some electronic claims. It is used on property/casualty/auto claims. This number is assigned by the property and casualty payer.

Policy Dates Start/End: Enter the beginning and ending dates of the policy. If the policy is still current, no date need be entered in the Stop field. This information is important when submitting claims to help ensure that the patient is actually covered at the time services are rendered. When a biller is making an appointment for the patient for a date in the future, this box should be checked to ensure that the patient still has insurance coverage on that date.

Assignment of Benefits/Accept Assignment: Does the provider accept Medicare Assignment on this patient? Place an X in the box for yes. Leave the box blank for no.

Capitated Plan: Is this patient a member of a capitated plan? If so, the provider receives a monthly payment that covers most services rendered to this

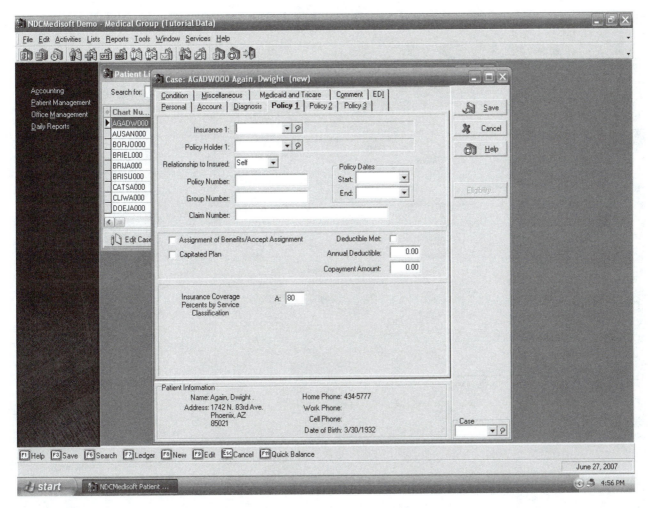

■ **Figure 6–7**   Policy 1 Screen

patient. If an X is entered in this box, the insurance coverage percent should indicate that the plan pays 100% of the charges. It is important for the biller to be aware of those charges that are not covered by the capitation amount and which charges should be billed on a fee-for-service basis. These items should be billed separately, under a separate case file. Normally services rendered that fall under the capitation plan will not require a bill to be generated; however, a record of procedures performed should be kept to assist the provider in understanding the cost of services rendered and in reporting to the carrier.

Deductible Met: Check this box if the patient has previously met their deductible. This field will help to determine the proper amount for the patient's portion of the visit.

Annual Deductible: Enter the amount of the patient's annual deductible. This field will also help to determine the proper amount for the patient's portion of the visit.

Copayment Amount: If the patient is part of a managed care plan that requires a copayment to be collected from the patient at the time of the visit, the copayment amount should be entered in this field. When entering charges in the Transaction Entry screen, this amount will appear at the bottom of the screen to remind you to collect these fees from the patient at the time of the visit.

Insurance Coverage Percents by Service Classification: Enter the standard coinsurance percentage that the insurance carrier pays. This information is used to calculate the estimated patient responsibility amount (i.e., on an 80/20 plan, the insurance covers 80% of the charge, and the patient is responsible for the other 20%). This amount will show up at the bottom of the Transaction Entry screen when charges are entered. Some providers prefer to have this amount collected from the patient at the time services are rendered, whereas others wait until the insurance carrier has paid their portion and then bill

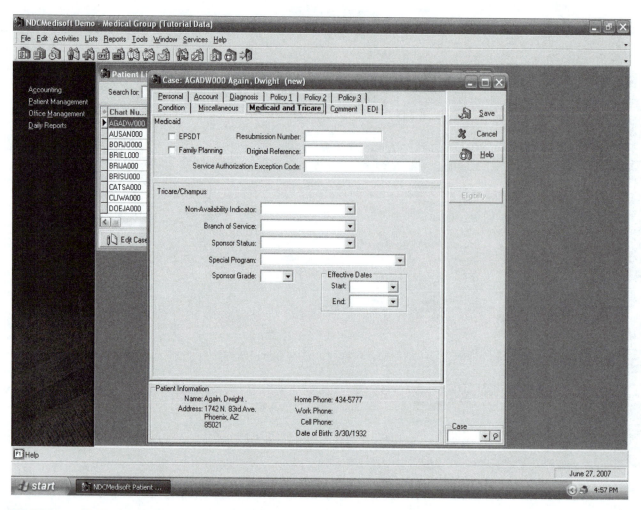

Figure 6–8   Medicaid and TRICARE Screen

the patient for any amounts not covered. However, MediSoft does not calculate any remaining deductible amount.

Policy 2 and Policy 3 Screens

The information in these screens is entered the same as for the Policy 1 screen discussed earlier. The Policy 2 screen is for the secondary payer, and the Policy 3 screen is for the tertiary payer. If there are no secondary or tertiary payers, these screens should be left blank.

Medicaid and TRICARE Screen

This screen is for entering information on Medicaid and TRICARE patients (**see Figure 6–8**).

EPSDT: The Early and Periodic Screening, Diagnosis, and Treatment program is intended to provide free or low-cost care to Medicaid infants. The attempt is to provide basic medical services to infants

to prevent a minor problem from becoming a major or lifelong one. Check this box if the service provided on this line is related to the EPSDT program.

21. Where does this information appear on a 1500 Health Insurance Claim form?

_____

Family Planning: If these services are related to family planning, check this box.

22. Where does this information appear on a 1500 Health Insurance Claim form?

_____

Resubmission/Original Reference Number: If Medicaid rejects a claim or sends it back for further information, often approval is required before resubmitting the claim. The Medicaid office will provide a resubmission number and an original reference number for the claim. These numbers should be entered in the appropriate boxes.

23. Where does this information appear on a 1500 Health Insurance Claim form?

_____

Service Authorization Exception Code: This code is required on some Medicaid claims. If you did not receive a service authorization code before seeing the patient, select one of the following codes:

1. Immediate/Urgent Care
2. Services Rendered in a Retroactive Period
3. Emergency Care
4. Client as Temporary Medicaid
5. Request from County for Second Opinion so Recipient Can Work
6. Request for Override Pending
7. Special Handling

TRICARE

This section is used for treating TRICARE patients at a nonmilitary facility or provider's location. Much of the information will be available on the patient's TRICARE card or from the patients themselves.

Nonavailability Indicator: Click on the ↓ to the right of this field to get a list of the choices indicated and enter one of the following indicators to show the patient's status:

- **NA statement obtained:** Nonavailability statement obtained. This indicates that there is no available military facility convenient to the patient and he/she therefore has permission to seek treatment at a nonmilitary facility.
- **NA statement not needed:** Nonavailability statement not needed.
- **Other carrier paid at least 75% of this claim**.

Or you may click on the ↓ to the right of this field to get a list of the choices indicated.

Branch of Service: Enter the appropriate branch of the military that the patient is connected with. Choices include the following:

- Air Force
- Army
- Champ VA (Veterans)
- Coast Guard
- Marines
- Navy
- Public Health Service
- National Oceanic and Atmospheric Administration (NOAA)

Sponsor Status: Enter one of the following to indicate the patient's military status.

- 100% Disabled
- Academy Student/Navy Officer Candidate School (OCS)
- Active
- Civilian
- Deceased
- Foreign Military
- Former Member
- Medal of Honor
- National Guard
- Other
- Permanently Disabled
- Recalled to Active Duty
- Reserves
- Retired
- Temporarily Disabled
- Unknown

Special Program: If applicable, a code can be entered to indicate a special program under which the patient is covered. Applicable codes are

- 03   Special Federal Funding
- 05   Disability
- 06   PPV/Medicare 100% Payment
- 07   Induced Abortion—Danger to Women's Life
- 08   Induced Abortion—Victim of Rape/Incest
- 09   Second Opinion/Surgery
- 30   Medicare demo proj. for lung surgery study
- A   Patient is sponsor
- B   Patient is spouse
- C1   Patient is child 1

- C2   Patient is child 2
- C3   Patient is child 3
- C4   Patient is child 4
- C5   Patient is child 5
- C6   Patient is child 6
- C7   Patient is child 7
- C8   Patient is child 8
- C9   Patient is child 9
- D   Patient is widow of sponsor
- 70   Local use*
- 71   Local use*
- 72   Local use*
- 73   Local use*
- 74   Local use*
- 75   Local use*
- 76   Local use*
- 77   Local use*
- 78   Local use*
- 79   Local use*
- 80   Local use*

*These codes are to be assigned by your local carrier.

Sponsor Grade: Enter the appropriate pay grade for the patient:

- W1–W4   Warrant Officer
- E1–E9   Enlisted
- 01–11   Officer
- VA   Civilian Health and Medical Program of the Department of Veterans Affairs (CHAMPVA)
- 19   Academy Student/Navy OCS
- 41–58   GS1–GS10
- G1   G1
- S1   S1
- 90   Unknown
- 99   Other

Effective Dates Start/End: Enter the date TRI-CARE coverage became effective as shown on the patient's TRICARE card and the date on which TRICARE coverage did or will terminate for this patient.

After entering the patient and case data, be sure to hit **F3** to save, or click the **Save** button. Your informa-tion will then be added to the Patient/Guarantor List, which will appear on the screen.

To exit the Patient/Guarantor screen, click on the **Close** button at the bottom of the screen.

Deleting A Patient

Before deleting a patient, you must be sure they have no current transactions, no outstanding balances, and no dependents.

If there are any current transactions, you will need to wait until after the next month-end processing. The month-end processing will move these transactions into history.

If there is an outstanding balance, it will need to be adjusted off. Determine whether there is an outstanding balance by printing a patient ledger. If there is an outstanding balance, you can enter an adjustment in the transaction entry screen to bring the balance to zero.

The preceding procedure should be done for each dependent and head of household before they are deleted. Then delete the dependents prior to deleting the head of household.

To delete a patient, go into the Patient List screen. You will automatically be entered into the search screen. Click on the patient or case you wish to delete and press **Delete Patient**. You will be asked to confirm that you want to delete this information. Click on either **Yes** or **No**.

It is possible to delete a specific case without deleting the information for the entire patient. To do this, simply click on the patient, and then click on the specific case you wish to delete prior to hitting the delete key.

If the patient still has transactions or outstanding balances, you may choose to place them on inactive status rather than deleting them. By clicking on the inactive button in the Patient Information screen, no new claims may be entered for this patient.

Printing A Patient Ledger

It is possible to print a patient ledger for a single patient while you are in the Patient Lists option. Highlight the patient and case you wish to print a ledger for and press **F7**, or click on the **F7** Ledger symbol at the bottom of the screen.

You can also print patient ledgers through the Reports Menu option.

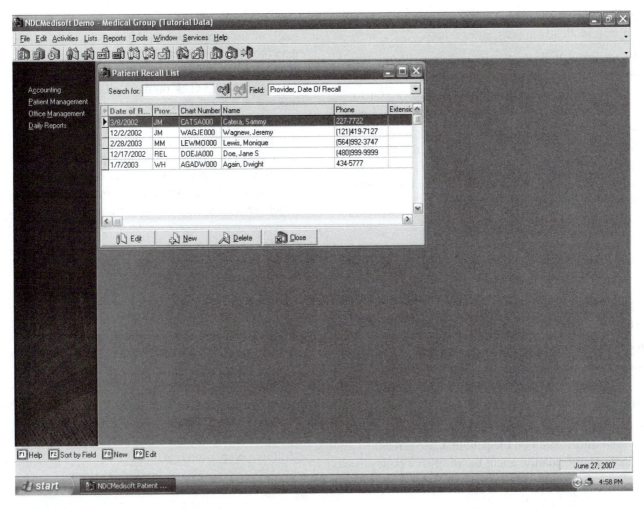

■ **Figure 6–9**   Patient Recall List

Patient Recall List

The **Patient Recall List (see Figure 6–9)** allows a practice to have a list of those patients who should be called for an additional appointment. This is most often used when the patient has a condition that necessitates a number of visits or continuous monitoring. For example, a patient with cancer in remission may need a visit and tests every six months to ensure that the cancer has not returned.

This list has the ability to be sorted by chart number, provider, or date. This allows the practice to print out a list of all the patients who should be recalled on a specific date, or patients who need to be scheduled for a visit with a specific provider.

To enter information on a patient who needs to be recalled, click on the Patient Recall Entry icon at the top of the screen or choose Patient Recall in the Lists menu and fill in the following fields:

Recall Date: Enter the date on which the patient should be recalled for a follow-up appointment.

Provider: Enter the code number for the provider the patient is to see. The provider must have been previously entered in the Provider List.

Chart: Enter the chart number of the patient. The patient must have previously been entered in the Patients/Guarantors List.

Name: If you entered a chart number in the preceding field, the name should automatically appear in this field. This allows you to have the name handy so that you can refer to the patient by name when you make the recall, rather than by chart number.

Phone: The phone number that was entered for the patient in the Patients/Guarantors list should appear here.

Extension: If the patient's extension number does not automatically appear, enter it here.

Procedure: Indicate the procedure code for the service for which the patient is being recalled. This is most often an office visit. This allows you to know the length of time a patient will need for an appointment.

Message: Indicate any message for the patient. This may be an explanation of why the patient is to follow up with the provider (i.e., to run tests to ensure that cancer has not returned).

Recall Status: These buttons allow you to keep track of the recall process. Upon first entering the data for a recall, the **Call** button will be highlighted. If you have called once and did not receive an answer, you would click on the **Call Again** button to indicate that at least one call was previously made to the patient. The **Appointment Set** button indicates that the call was successful and an appointment has been set for this patient. The **No Appointment** button indicates that you were successful in reaching the patient and spoke with them; however, the patient refused to set up an appointment at that time.

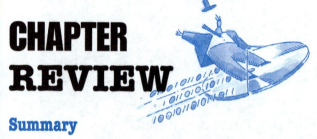

CHAPTER REVIEW

Summary

- The Patients/Guarantors screens contain personal information on the patient. Case screens include information about the insurance policy covering the patient, the condition for which they are being treated, and their account. Most screens will only need to be updated when information changes; however, the Condition screen should be checked each time a patient visits the doctor and before billing on a 1500 Health Insurance Claim form.

- MediSoft also has a Recall List in the List Menu, which allows you to keep track of all patients who need to be contacted regarding a follow-up appointment.

Questions for Review

Directions: Answer the following questions without looking back into the material just covered. Write your answers in the space provided.

1. List the four categories used for setting up case files.

    1. _____

    _____

    2. _____

    _____

    3. _____

    _____

    4. _____

    _____

2. What is the purpose of having case-based files?

_____

_____

_____

3. What is the purpose of the Patient Recall List?

_____

_____

4. Before deleting a patient you must be sure they have no _____

_____, _____ or _____

_____

5. What does the EDI/EMC notes window allow?

_____

_____

_____

If you were unable to answer any of the questions, refer back to that section, and then fill in the answers.

7

Activities Menu Options

After completion of this chapter
you will be able to:

- Enter charge, payment, and adjustment transactions into the MediSoft system.
- Create, edit, print/reprint, and send claims for transactions that you have entered.

The Activities menu option allows you to Enter Transactions, perform Claims Management, and use the Appointment Book. Most activities involving the patient occur in the Enter Transactions screen. The Appointment Entry screen in the Appointment Book is used to enter appointments. Because the Appointment Book option opens an entirely new computer program called the MediSoft Office Hours program, it will be discussed in its own chapter (Chapter 10).

Transaction Entry

All charges, adjustments, payments, copayments, credits, lab charges, and general comments are entered into the patient's record through the Transaction Entry screen **(see Figure 7–2).**

Go back to the information entered in the Procedure/Payment/Adjustment Code List to see the types of entries that are available using this screen. Each of the options entered in the procedure information screen will be added to a patient chart through the Enter Transactions screen. This screen is the one most often used by the medical biller during the course of normal operations.

Exercise **7-1**

Pat N. O'Gen saunters up to the billing office window after her son's visit with Dr. Sickman. Create a family and patient chart. Enter these charges into the system.

Ox O'Gen received a problem-focused, straightforward visit performed in the office ($55) today (date of first visit 12/29/PY). Diagnosis: Scarlet Fever, Upper Respiratory Infection (URI).

As you read through the following information, enter this charge into the system.

Also remember that information concerning the patient's condition may need to be added in the Patient Information record, and the Condition Screen.

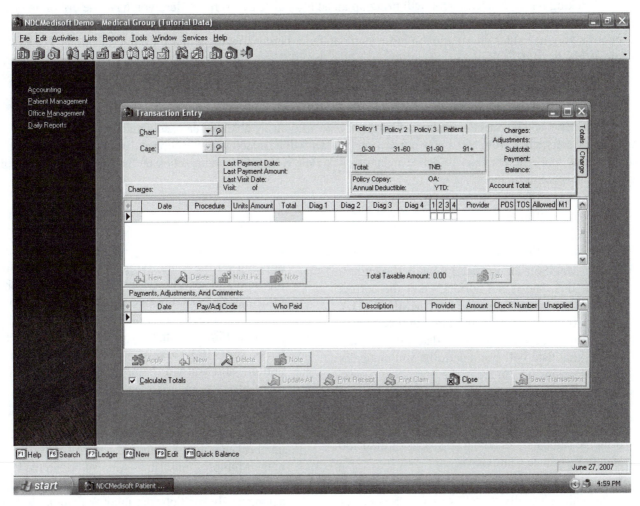

■ **Figure 7–1** Transaction Entry Screen

You may need to look up the procedures and diagnoses in the CPT® and ICD-9-CM books. These codes will be entered during the entry of this patient's charges if they were not previously entered in the Procedure/Payment/Adjustments List and Diagnosis List screens.

Chart: Enter the patient's chart number. If you do not know the patient's full chart number, this box has an automatic search feature. Simply begin entering the chart number, and the first matching entry will pop up on the screen. This feature will bring up every chart number that matches the characteristics of the data you entered. If there is more than one choice, they will be listed in a search screen. If there is only one match to your entry, the chart number for that person will appear on the screen. If you do not know the chart number, you may search for the patient by pressing **F6** or clicking on the magnifying glass icon.

Once a patient chart number has been chosen, the patient's name and birth date will appear to the right of the chart number. This can help to ensure that you have chosen the correct patient.

Case: Enter the number for the case of treatment to which these entries will be associated. It is important to match the transaction entries with the correct case scenario to correctly bill and apply transactions and payments. If only one case has been entered for this patient, it will appear in this field, and the diagnosis will appear to the right of the field.

Briefcase Icon: To the right of the case field is a briefcase icon. This icon allows you to search for a case by a transaction date, procedure code, or amount. This can be very helpful when an insurance carrier has made a payment on a claim. The Explanation of Benefits (EOB) often will not list the diagnosis. Therefore, by matching either the transaction date, procedure code, or amount, you can find the correct case file. This can be very important because you must be in the proper case file for payments to be properly posted to their charges.

Clicking on the briefcase icon will bring up an additional search screen. Here you have the option to enter a date in the **Date From** field, a procedure code in the **Code** field, or an amount in the **Amount** field. If you choose, you may enter information in more than one field. Doing so will further limit the selections. For example, if you have an EOB that lists an office visit on a specific date, along with several other procedures, entering both a date and a procedure will further help the MediSoft program to choose the correct case that the payment applies to.

In the Charge and Payment/Adjustment Comment Screens, you are able to create, edit, and delete transactions. To create a new entry, click **New,** and a new transaction field set will be added with the current date. You may change the date by typing in a different date. To delete an entry, click **Delete**. To edit an entry, click on the field you wish to edit and enter the new information.

Charge Entry Screen

Dates: MediSoft automatically enters the current date. If this date is not correct, enter the correct date of the charge (service) in the MMDDCCYY format. If there is a from and through date associated with the service, enter both dates. If you enter a date, that date will continue to be automatically entered as long as you are in the Enter New Transactions screen. This allows you to enter all charges from a certain day without reentering the date each time. If only one date is entered, MediSoft will print the same date in both date spaces of the 1500 Health Insurance Claim form.

Procedure: Enter the appropriate procedure code. This is usually a CPT® or HCPCS code for a medical procedure. If you do not know the code, it can be looked up by pressing **F6** or by clicking on the magnifying glass to the right of the field and searching for the information. If the information has not been entered in the Procedure Code List screen, you may access this screen by pressing **F8.** Once the information has been entered, press **F3** to save (or click on the **Save** button), and you will be returned to the Transaction Entry screen.

Units: Enter the number of days, times, or units this service was provided. The default setting is 1. If a number other than 1 is entered and you placed an X in the Multiply Units Times Amount box in the Program Options (File/Program Options), MediSoft will automatically multiply the number of units by the amount and enter the result in the Amount column.

1. Where on the 1500 Health Insurance Claim form will the number of units show up?

_____

_____

Amount: If the Procedure code listed was a CPT® code, MediSoft will automatically enter the amount for the procedure that was entered into the Procedure Code List. If this default amount is incorrect or is unavailable, type in the new amount.

Total: The total amount of the transactions will appear here. If the system is not set up to automatically multiply the units by the amount, you may need to enter the total amount in this field.

Diag 1/2/3/4: Enter the diagnosis code(s) for this episode of treatment. This is especially important when billing for charges, as insurance carriers will not pay claims where no diagnosis is indicated. MediSoft allows you to enter up to four diagnosis codes. If there are more diagnosis codes, the transaction entries should be split. Enter all transactions that correspond to one, two, three, or four diagnoses on one screen, save the data, and then enter the additional procedures for any remaining diagnoses on a separate entry.

Diagnosis Boxes 1, 2, 3, and 4: Place a ✓; in the box for each diagnosis that relates to this procedure. The applicable diagnoses were entered in the upper-right corner of the screen.

Provider: Enter the code for the physician who provided this service to the patient. The default setting is the Assigned Provider that was entered in the Patient Information screen.

POS (Place of Service): This code indicates the location where the procedure was performed. For a complete listing, see the 1500 Health Insurance Claim form instructions or the back of many 1500 forms. If you listed a default location code in the Procedure List screen, this code will automatically appear in this space. If it is incorrect, change it by typing in the new location code.

TOS (Type of Service): Enter the type of service for this charge/procedure. This field is often left blank.

Allowed: This field lists the Medicare allowed amount for this procedure.

MultiLink: If you want to enter a MultiLink code, click on the MultiLink button. This will bring up a new screen that allows you to enter the MultiLink code.

M1/M2/M3 (Modifiers): Enter the modifiers, if any, associated with this procedure.

NOTE: If there are any notes to be associated with this claim, enter them here.

Payments/Adjustments/Comments Entry Screen

The Payments/Adjustments/Comments Entry screen allows you to enter payments, adjustments, and comments that have been made on a patient's account.

Exercise 7-2

Pat. N. O'Gen is still at the window. "I would like to make a payment on the bill I just got."

She takes out her checkbook and hands you check #2929, bank #22-31, in the amount of $25. See claim 1 in the Window Payments section. Enter this payment in the Transaction Entry screen.

Date: MediSoft automatically enters the current date. If this date is not correct, enter the correct date of the payment in the MMDDCCYY format.

Pay/Adj Code: Enter the appropriate code for the type of payment or adjustment. These codes should previously have been entered using the Procedures/Payments/Adjustments List screen. The Pay/Adj Code alerts MediSoft as to whether this is a payment or an adjustment.

Who Paid: Enter the name of the person who made this payment. Clicking on the ↓ to the right of this field will bring up several options. If you are unable to find the correct person, it means they have not been entered in the Patient/Guarantor List or Insurance List. They will need to be entered before they can be placed in this field.

Description: If the procedure was a payment by check, enter the check number, followed by the bank number (i.e., ck #1099, 16-999). If the procedure was an adjustment, enter the reason for the adjustment. For example, if you incorrectly coded a claim, enter incorrect coding and include the incorrect code along with the new, corrected code. This information is necessary when providers' accounts are audited.

Provider: Enter the code for the physician who provided this service to the patient. The default setting is the Assigned Provider that was entered into the Patient Information screen.

Amount: Enter the amount of the payment. MediSoft automatically recognizes that this is a payment and subtracts all payments from charges. Therefore, a minus (–) sign in front of the amount is not necessary. Because Adjustments can be either a credit (added to the account) or a debit (subtracted from the account), enter a minus sign in front of the amount for debit adjustments.

Check Number: Enter the check number here.

Unapplied: If the amount of the check is greater than the amount owed, there will be an unapplied amount. The program will automatically calculate this amount.

Apply: The Apply button applies payment to the charges. This does not appear in all versions of MediSoft.

Previous Versions of MediSoft

In previous versions of MediSoft, the Payment and Adjustment entries had two separate screens. The information that goes in each field is still the same.

Document: This is one of the most important numbers in the Transaction Entry screen. This number is used to tie all charges and payments together. Therefore it is vitally important that this number be the same for all entries that relate to each other. For example, if a patient is seen by the doctor on 10/1/CCYY and incurs charges of $500, the document number for the charges, the insurance payment, the patient payment, and any write-off should all carry the same document number. This allows you to see how much is outstanding on each bill, rather than just on the account as a whole.

A document number may be an invoice number, a date, a charge number, or any other number the practice chooses. MediSoft automatically enters the current date in the YYMMDD format. For purposes of this book, we will use the date of services as the document number.

Apply Payments to Charges: This field allows you to apply the payment to the correct charge. For example, a patient may be treated for a fractured leg, and their insurance covers procedures, but does not cover durable medical equipment (i.e., crutches). They may want to make a payment on the crutches but want to wait until the insurance carrier has paid before making a payment on the visit.

When each entry has been completed, you are ready to end the transaction. The icons on the right of the transaction screen allow you to perform the following functions (the keystrokes in parentheses can also be used to complete the function):

1. Saves this transaction and then opens a new transaction (Shift **F3**); this function is used when you have additional transactions to enter.

2. Saves this transaction and closes the new transaction panel (**F3**); this function is used when you are finished entering transactions for this patient.

3. Abandon any changes or entries without saving.

4. Enter Transaction Documentation. This is a screen in which you are able to type notes regarding this transaction. These notes are used to substantiate services or to reflect information that should be known regarding these procedures. This screen can be especially important when submitting electronic claims because this is the only additional documentation that can be sent to substantiate the medical necessity of services. You are allowed up to 255 characters. There are eight types of Transaction Documentation:

   1. Operative Note: A note to substantiate the cause of operation.

   2. Other: Miscellaneous notes that are important for correct processing of this claim.

   3. Oxygen Prescription: A prescription for oxygen therapy or equipment.

   4. PEN Certification: Prescription for parenteral therapy. Physical Therapy Certification: Notes to substantiate the need for physical therapy services.

   5. Physical Therapy Certification: Notes to substantiate the need for physical therapy services.

6. Prosthetics/Orthotics Certification: A prescription for prosthetic or orthotic equipment, or notes to substantiate the need for such services.

7. Statement Note: A note that appears on the patient statement to explain additional charges, adjustments, etc.

8. Transaction Note: A note that is generated for internal use only and will not appear on the claim forms submitted to the carrier.

Transaction Entry Screen Display

In the upper-right-hand corner is a pair of boxes that summarizes some of the information for this and previous transactions to assist in properly billing the patient. It contains information about the patient and their account.

Last Visit Date and Visit # of #: If the insurance carrier authorized a series of visits for this patient (i.e., 10 chiropractic visits for a back injury), these fields will display the date of the last visit and the number of visits that have been completed. It will also show the number of visits that were authorized. This allows you to warn the patient if they are nearing the end of the number of visits authorized.

Last Payment Date and Last Payment Amount: These fields display the date and amount of the last payment made on this patient. This information is taken from all previous entries in the transaction screen.

Estimated Responsibility Amounts (Policy 1, 2, 3): MediSoft will automatically calculate the estimated insurance payment by each payer, based on the information entered in the Insurance List. For example, if the patient had only one insurance carrier and they covered all procedures at 80%, then 80% of the charges entered would be shown in this space.

Guarantor: This field shows the estimated amount of the guarantor's responsibility (i.e., the remaining 20% that the insurance does not cover). Any deductible not paid, allowed amounts, or other items that may affect payment are not calculated into either the Insurance or Patient Share fields.

Adjustments: This field shows any adjustments that have been entered on this account.

Policy Copay: The amount of copayment is shown here. This is the amount that should be collected from the patient at the time services are rendered. If a copayment is required from the patient and you attempt to save and exit the Transaction Entry screen without entering a copayment amount, a reminder notice will appear. This reminder notice gives you the option of returning to the entry screen and entering the copayment amount, or saving without collecting the copayment.

Annual Deductible and **YTD:** This field pulls the annual insurance deductible from **Case** window, Policy 1 tab. The **YTD** field calculates how much of the deductible the patient has paid.

OA: Other Arrangements. If anything had been entered in the Other Arrangements field of the Patients/Guarantors List, that information would show up here. This is to remind you of any special arrangements that may have been made on this account (i.e., professional courtesy, no charge).

Charges: This field shows the total of all charges entered at this time.

Adjustments: This field shows the total of all adjustments entered at this time.

Subtotal: This field shows a subtotal of the charges and adjustments entered at this time.

Payment: This field shows a total of all payments entered at this time.

Balance: This field shows the result of the subtotal minus the payments.

Account Total: This field shows the result of the balance, plus any remaining balance that was previously shown on this account.

Once you have finished entering transactions you have five options:

1. Update All: will update all transactions entered.
2. Print Receipt: will print the patient a walkout receipt for the charges and payments just entered.
3. Print Claim: will print a 1500 Health Insurance Claim form using all entries that have not yet been placed on a claim.
4. Close: will close the transaction window.
5. Save Transactions: will save your input.

Claim Management

The Claim Management screen allows you to select claims that you wish to print or send electronically, reprint, edit, or delete. The first step is to choose the claims that you wish to perform one of the preceding functions on. Any claims must have previously been entered in the Transaction Entry screen.

Create Claims Screen

Begin by clicking on the **Create Claims (see Figure 7–2)** button on the bottom of the claim management screen. This will bring up the Create Claims screen. Choose the transactions you wish to incorporate on a claim by setting the following parameters.

Transaction Dates: Enter the beginning and ending dates of the transactions you wish to work with. You may also click on the calendar to choose a date. This can be helpful if you are unsure of the number of days in a month (i.e., 30 or 31).

Chart Numbers: Enter the beginning and ending chart numbers of the transactions you wish to work with. If you are unsure of the chart numbers, you may click on the magnifying glass to search for a specific number. If you wish to work with

only one chart number, enter the same number in both the beginning and ending fields.

Select Transactions That Match: This section allows you to be more specific in your parameters.

Primary Insurance: Enter the Insurance Carrier code. You can enter multiple codes by placing a comma between each code. Leave the space blank to indicate all carriers.

Billing Codes: Enter the billing code. You can enter multiple billing codes by placing a comma between each code. Leave the space blank to indicate all codes.

Case Indicator: Enter the case indicator (i.e., case 1). You can enter multiple case indicators by placing a comma between each one. Leave the space blank to indicate all case indicators.

Location: Enter the location code (place where services were performed). You can enter multiple location codes by placing a comma between each one. Leave the space blank to indicate all location codes.

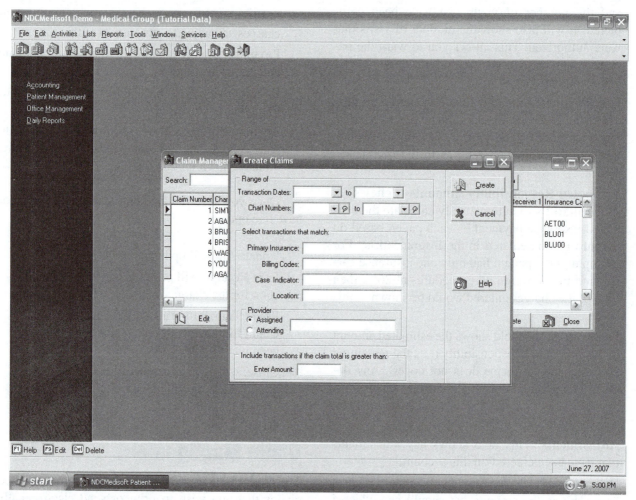

■ Figure 7–2 Create Claims

Provider: Enter the provider code. You can enter multiple provider codes by placing a comma between each one. Leave the space blank to indicate all providers. Indicate whether the provider is Assigned or Attending.

Include transactions if the sum is greater than: This option allows you to create claims for transactions with a specific minimum total dollar amount.

Enter amount: Enter a minimum total amount for a case.

Once you have chosen the parameters, MediSoft will take all transactions that meet these parameters and lump them together on a claim. Therefore, if you have chosen to create a claim for one patient, and that patient has current transactions, but also previous transactions that have not yet been billed, MediSoft will place all open transactions on a single claim and bill them together.

Because of this, it is important that you create claims that match each other. For example, if a patient has two cases, one for a workers' compensation injury and one for their regular treatment, you will need to first create a claim for their regular treatment and then create a new claim for their workers' compensation treatment because you cannot bill for both types of services on the same claim.

Once you have created the claim(s), you may choose to perform one of the following functions:

1. Edit the information on the claim by clicking on the **Edit** button.
2. Print a paper claim and/or send an electronic claim.
3. Reprint the claim.
4. Delete the claim.

Edit Claim Icon Option

This option allows you to change data on the claim you have already created. There are five types of changes you can make:

1. Changes to the information for carrier 1.
2. Changes to the information for carrier 2.
3. Changes to the information for carrier 3.
4. Changes to the transaction.
5. Add comments to the claim.

Carrier 1, 2, and 3 Screens

These screens are used for entering information on the insurance carrier.

Claim Status: These fields help to track each claim. Once a claim has been completed with all appropriate information, the computer will mark it "Ready to Send." If you wish to change the status of the claim, you may do so here. Your choices are

Hold the claim to Print/Send at a future date.

Ready to Send.

Sent (once a claim has been sent electronically, the MediSoft program will indicate this). If you are printing claims and sending them in on paper, you will need to manually click on this item when a claim has been sent.

Rejected indicates that the claim was rejected by the insurance carrier or by the clearinghouse.

Challenge indicates that you are or will be appealing the rejection of the claim.

Alert is used to indicate when something is wrong on the claim, and further research may need to be done (i.e., no word has been received from the insurance carrier for an extended period of time).

Done indicates that the claim has been paid by the insurance carrier. Some offices will not mark a claim as done until the patient has paid their portion of the claim, and the claim has a zero balance.

Pending indicates that the claim is being held until further information is received from the provider or the patient.

Billing Method: This section allows you to choose whether to send a claim on paper or electronically. For example, if you normally send claims electronically, you may want to print out and send manually a claim that needs several pages of documentation.

Batch/Submission Count: The MediSoft program will automatically batch together claims that are sent and will indicate the batch number here, along with the number of claims included in the batch.

Billing Date: This box allows you to indicate the date on which these claims were billed. This can help track how long it has been since a claim was submitted and whether or not you need to follow up with the insurance carrier.

Insurance 1: This box will indicate the primary insurance carrier associated with this claim(s).

EDI/EMC Receiver: This box allows you to change the entity (i.e., clearinghouse) that will be receiving this claim.

Transactions Screen

This screen allows you to edit the transactions that appear on this claim.

Comment Screen

This screen allows you to add a comment or additional documentation regarding this claim or the sending of this claim.

Print/Send Claims Icon Option

This option allows you to print paper claims and/or send electronic claims. Upon clicking on the choice, you will be given the option of printing paper claims or sending electronic claims. Only one choice may be done at a time. If you are choosing to send electronic claims, you may choose the receiver to whom you are

sending the claims. If you are sending claims to more than one receiver, you will need to complete the sending of claims to one receiver, and then choose to print claims for a second receiver.

Often provider offices will choose to send claims to only one clearinghouse. However, even if a clearinghouse has been chosen, there may be a few insurance carriers who wish to have claims submitted directly to them.

Reprint Claim Icon Option

This screen allows you to reprint a claim that has already been printed. Upon clicking on this choice, you will be asked for the proper format of the claim you wish to reprint or the carrier you wish to reprint the claim for. This choice is most often used when there are several carriers on a claim, and you need to print a separate claim for each carrier, or when a claim has been lost or misplaced and needs to be resubmitted.

Delete Claim Icon Option

This will delete a claim that you have just created. Thus, any transactions that were associated with this claim will be released, and you may then choose to create a different claim using these transactions.

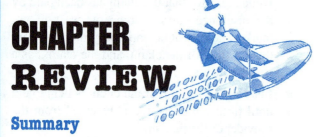

CHAPTER REVIEW

Summary

- The Activities Menu option includes the Enter Transaction screens and the Claim Management screens. Most activities involving the patient occur in the Transaction Entry screen. This is where all charges, payments, and adjustments are entered into the system. The Claim Management screens allow you to create and print or send claims as well as edit the claims.

Questions for Review

Directions: Answer the following questions without looking back into the material just covered. Write your answers in the space provided.

1. What items are entered through the Transaction Entry screen?

_____

_____

2. List two reasons you want to reprint a claim.

1. _____

2. _____

3. How do you end an entry in the Charge Entry screen?

_____

_____

4. What are the five types of changes you can make to a claim you have created?

1. _____

2. _____

3. _____

4. _____

5. _____

5. Once you have finished entering transactions, what are your five options?

1. _____

2. _____

3. _____

4. _____

5. _____

If you were unable to answer any of the questions, refer back to that section, and then fill in the answers.

8
Reports Menu Options

After completion of this chapter
you will be able to:

- Identify and create various reports.
- Print reports.

The Reports Menu option allows you to print reports to assist in the running of the office and analyzing the practice's accounts. It includes options such as printing patient day sheets; procedure day sheets; payments day sheets; patient ledgers; patient aging; practice analysis; primary, secondary, and tertiary insurance aging; and patient statements. There is also an option for custom reports (i.e., patient lists, address lists, etc.) and for designing your own reports and bills.

Upon choosing many of the options in this list, you will be presented with a window that asks "Print Report Where?" Your three selections are

1. Preview the report on the screen.
2. Print the report on the printer.
3. Export the report to a file.

Choose the option you prefer. If desired, you can preview the report on the screen and then print it to the printer.

Once you have chosen one of the print options, click on **Start** to begin the printing process or **Cancel** to take you out of the Reports Menu. If you choose Start, you will be taken into a second screen that allows you to set the parameters for the reports by asking certain questions.

Sort Questions

Because most options present you with the same screen, we will list the questions that may appear on the various screens, then describe each screen and its purpose. These questions help to limit the report to the items you want, rather than including everything. Note that if you do not enter any information in the given field, it indicates there is no limitation for the search, and all records will be included.

Some fields will appear on some screens, but not others. Additionally, some of these fields will appear on some versions of MediSoft, but not others. To print reports, simply complete the fields found in your version, and then choose the option to print.

Chart Number Range: Enter the range of the chart numbers you wish to print. Chart numbers are sorted alphabetically. Pressing Enter will include all chart numbers. If you wish to print a ledger for a single person, enter the patient's chart number in both the beginning and ending positions (i.e., ANDAD010–ANDAD010).

Date Created Range: Enter the "from" and "to" dates for which the report was created.

Date From Range: Enter the beginning and ending dates that you want included on the report. These can include the date the reports were created or date of service on claims.

Attending Provider Range: Enter the range of provider codes for the providers you would like included in this report. Providers are chosen according to their placement in the Provider List. Pressing Enter will include all providers.

Patient Billing Code Range: If you only wish to include patients within certain billing codes, enter the range of billing codes here. This item corresponds with the Billing Codes that were entered in the Billing Codes List. This allows you to limit patients to those in a certain billing cycle or billed during a certain time of month. To include all patients, press **Enter**.

Patient Indicator Match: This field refers to the Patient Indicator field that was used in the Patient Information Account screen. Using patient indicators in conjunction with billing codes can create a wide range of printing possibilities. For example, if you wanted to indicate all patients with a certain diagnosis, this diagnosis could be used as an indicator. Thus, you could print all patients with a certain diagnosis who are billed during the first week of the month.

Code 1 Range: Enter the range of the codes from the Procedure/Payment/Adjustments List that you would like included in the report. This option allows you to limit your report to certain types of procedures. For example, entering 99201 to 99215 will limit the report to all office visits.

Patient Reference Balance Range: This field allows you to limit the report to only those patients who have an outstanding balance on their account. Enter the beginning and ending range of the balances you would like to print with no decimal or cents amount. For example, you may want to print only those patients who have a balance of more than $5 but less than $100 (i.e., 5–100). To print $5 and above, enter 5 to 999999. If you leave this field blank, the report will show all families, whether they have current transactions and balances or not.

Insurance Carrier 1, 2, or 3 Range: Enter a range of insurance carrier codes. The code refers to the insurance code entered in the Insurance Information screen. The 1, 2, or 3 indicates whether the carriers pay as primary, secondary, or tertiary on the claim.

Primary/Secondary Billing Date Range: Enter the beginning and ending dates you want included on the report. Primary refers to the first date for which the claim was billed. Secondary refers to the date this claim was first submitted to the secondary insurance carrier.

Patient Type Range: Enter the types of patients you would like included in the report. These patients can be sorted to include only those covered by Medicare, Medicaid, or group insurance.

Preview Screen Icons

Once you preview a report on the screen, a new set of icons will appear across the top of the page. These icons can help you to view the report more easily and to move quickly among the different pages of a report. The presence of certain icons will depend on which version of MediSoft you are using.

The report can be shown in three different sizes on the screen. To change the size of the report, click on one of the first three icons at the top left of the page.

The **first icon** will make the report fit within the size of your screen. The **second icon** will enlarge the picture to 100% of what would print.

Because most screens are less than 8.5 by 11 inches, this means that a portion of the report will be off the sides and the top or bottom of the screen.

The **third icon** will enlarge the report so that its width is the same width as your screen. This allows you to see more detail, but some items will be scrolled off the top or the bottom of the page.

The **navigation keys** will move you through the various pages of the reports. The first one will return you to the first page in the document. The second one will move you back one page. The third one will move you forward one page, and the last one will move you to the last page of the report. Most appointment lists for a single doctor have only one page, so these items are not always used with the appointment menu.

The **Printer icon** allows you to print reports from the screen to the printer.

The **Diskette icon** will save the report to a diskette.

The **Close icon** will exit you from the report preview screen.

The **Go To Page box** `Goto Page: 1` will allow you to move to a specified page quickly by entering the page number you wish to appear on the screen.

Following are descriptions of each of the different reports and options found under the Reports Menu option.

Day Sheets

A day sheet gives an overview of the provider's day. The **Patient Day Sheet** details the patients seen, showing all transactions and a summary of the day's activities. The **Procedure Day Sheet** details the procedures that were done and shows the patient treated for each procedure. The **Payment Day Sheet** details the money the practice received on that day broken into cash payments, copayments, check payments, and insurance payments and shows the charges to which the payments were applied.

Patient Ledger

A patient ledger records all transactions on a patient's account. It shows the services received, billed amounts, payments, adjustments, and balances. It is useful in noting the activity on each patient's account.

With MediSoft, you can include only those transactions that have not been paid or all transactions for a given range of dates.

Exercise 8-1

Print a patient ledger for Ben Waite. Accept the default setting for all selection questions except Attending Provider Range. Here, you will include only Dr. Phil Goode's patients. Enter the provider code for Dr. Phil Goode in both range areas.

1. What information is included on the patient ledger?

_____

_____

_____

Patient Aging

A patient aging report allows you to see which patients have outstanding balances and the length of time those balances have been outstanding. This report is most often used when attempting to collect on past due accounts. MediSoft calculates the number of days between the creation of the transaction or claim and the date of the report. The columns break down into 30, 60, 90, and 90+ days old. Because this report is taken from the date the transaction was created (not the date services were rendered), it gives a more accurate picture of how long an account has had an open balance on it. For this reason it is important to enter transactions and create claims as soon after the services were rendered as possible.

Exercise **8-2**

Print a patient aging report for all patients with balances. Include only Dr. Phil Goode's clients.

2. List some of the items included on a Patient Aging Report.

_____

_____

_____

_____

_____

_____

Practice Analysis

This report prints the procedures done during a specified period, the amount charged, quantity performed, and the costs and net amount received for each code. It allows the practice to see the types of procedures they are performing and the net receipts from those services. Some practices use this report in creating their monthly financial statements.

Exercise **8-3**

Print a practice analysis with all procedure codes, dates, and providers.

3. What information is included on the Practice Analysis Report?

_____

_____

_____

Primary/Secondary/Tertiary Insurance Aging

Insurance Aging Reports allow a practice to see the age of those claims that have been submitted to insurance carriers for payment. Reports are sorted by insurance carrier, thus allowing a biller to see all claims that are owed by a single carrier. Patients who have both primary and secondary insurance will appear on two reports, one for each carrier. As with the Patient Aging Report, Insurance Aging Reports calculate the age of the claim by the number of days between the time the transaction was entered and the date the report was printed. Entries are then separated into 30, 60, 90, 120, and 120+ columns.

Below each patient listed, a tally line appears showing the totals in each aging column both for that patient and for the insurance carrier. The insurance carrier's portion is calculated by multiplying the patient's amount times the percentage of insurance coverage (i.e., 80% in an 80/20 plan).

Exercise 8-4

View on the screen an insurance aging report for all primary insurances. Include all dates and all providers.

4. List some of the items included on an Insurance Aging Report.

_____

_____

_____

_____

Patient Statements

Patient Statements are sent to patients every month to give them a record of their visits and the payments on those visits. They are used by many practices as a monthly bill for patients.

MediSoft allows you several different types of patient statements:

- Patient Statement (30, 60, 90)

- Patient Statement (Color)
- Patient Statement (Color) (30, 60, 90)
- Patient Statement (with charges only)
- Preprinted Statement (with text only, so you can use a preprinted form)
- Sample Statement with Image and a Sample Statement with Logo.

You are also given the option of showing file names.

Exercise 8-5

Preview patient statements on the screen. Choose the Patient Statement report title (not color or preprinted). Choose all charts, dates, billing code ranges, indicator ranges, and patient types. It may take a moment to generate this report. After viewing the report, print the statement for Ben Waite by going to the page showing his statement. Click on the printer icon at the top of the screen. Choose the Pages Print Range and enter the page number for Ben Waite's statement (from the upper-right corner of the screen).

5. List some of the items included on a Patient Statement.

_____

_____

_____

Custom Report List

MediSoft has created a number of custom reports. Most of these include lists of the data entered into the Lists menu option. These lists have been created by MediSoft. To print a list, click on the type of list you would like to print, and then click on **OK**.

Exercise 8-6

Print a Patient List for all patients in the practice.

6. What information is included on a Patient List?

_____

_____

_____

_____

_____

_____

Load Saved Reports: This option allows you to reopen reports that were prepared earlier and were saved.

Design Custom Reports and Bills

With this option, MediSoft allows you to create your own customized reports and bills. Each practice can design a specific report, letter, or document with data imported from the lists or any specific portion of the list. If you wish to create a customized report, consult your MediSoft Patient Accounting User Manual.

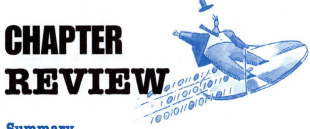

CHAPTER REVIEW

Summary

- The Reports Menu option allows you to print reports to assist in the running of the office and analyzing the practice's accounts. It includes options such as printing patient day sheets; procedure day sheets; payment day sheets, patient ledgers; patient aging, practice analysis; primary, secondary, and tertiary insurance aging; and patient statements. There is also an option for custom reports (i.e., patient lists, address lists, etc.) and for designing your own reports and bills.
- For each report, you have the option of displaying the report on the screen or printing it to paper.

Questions for Review

Directions: Answer the following questions without looking back into the material just covered. Write your answers in the space provided.

1. What information is included on the Patient Ledger?

_____

_____

_____

2. What is the purpose of the Insurance Aging Report?

_____

_____

_____

_____

3. What information is included on a Patient Day Sheet?

_____

_____

4. What information is included on a Practice Analysis?

_____

_____

_____

_____

5. How do you preview a report on the screen?

_____

_____

_____

If you were unable to answer any of the questions, refer back to that section, and then fill in the answers.

9

Edit, Tools, Window, and Help Menus

After completion of this chapter
you will be able to:

- Demonstrate use of the Edit and Tools menu options.
- Access the Help menu to assist in using the MediSoft program.

The items within the Edit, Tools, Window, and Help Menus are not as extensive as those in previously mentioned Menus, and thus we will deal with all of them in this chapter.

Edit Menu Options

The Edit Menu option deals primarily with the handling of text, often in specific windows. By using your mouse to highlight a portion of the text, you may choose to perform any of the following options. To highlight a portion of text, use your mouse to position the cursor at the beginning of the text that you wish to cut, copy, or delete. Then, while holding down the left mouse button, move the cursor to the end of the text you wish to modify. Once the text is highlighted, choose one of the following options:

Cut the highlighted portion of the text. This is most often done when you wish to move a portion of the text from one area to another. To move text you would first highlight it, and then click on **Cut**. You would then move the cursor to where you wish to insert the text and use the paste option.

Copy the highlighted portion of the text. This will leave the selected text in its original location and also copy it to the new location of your choice. First highlight the portion of the text you wish to copy. Then click on the **Copy** option. Then move your cursor to the position where you wish the text to be copied and use the paste option.

Paste the highlighted portion of the text. This option inserts the portion of text that was last cut into the current position of the cursor.

Delete the highlighted portion of the text. Once a portion of text has been highlighted, by clicking on this option, the highlighted portion of the text will be erased.

Using these options will allow you to modify your text faster than if you were to use the delete keys and/or type in the information again.

Tools Menu Options

The Tools Menu option allows you to look up information regarding your system and its setup, as well as to use an on-screen calculator.

The **Calculator** within the MediSoft system works the same as a normal desktop calculator. It can perform addition, subtraction, multiplication, and division functions, as well as calculate percents and square roots. You can use your numeric keypad to enter numbers and operations into the calculator (with the Num Lock on), or you can use your mouse to choose numbers and functions. This tool can be especially useful when performing transaction entries.

The **NDCMediSoft™ Terminal** menu option can be used to send or receive various reports by connecting to various bulletin boards using a modem. A Bulletin Board System (BBS) is a system that can provide you with information regarding the status of your claims. Because we are not equipped to send claims electronically, we will not be using this option.

The **View File** option allows you to open and view an existing file that has previously been saved.

The **Add/Copy User Reports** option allows you to add or copy reports that you have created.

The **Collection Letter Wizard** option allows you to create a collections letter by just inputting the patient's information.

The **Customize Menu Bars** option allows you to change the icons that appear on your system or the menu bars that appear at the side of your screen.

Choosing the **System Information** option will bring up information regarding your system, including which version of Windows and DOS you are using, how much space you have available in your computer, and the type of printer you are using. This screen is for informational purposes only. Nothing can be edited here.

The **Modem Check** option allows you to test your modem to see if it is working. Because we are not sending items electronically, we will not be using this menu option.

The **User Information** option creates a User Information Report. This report details the name and address of the practice, its phone number, and tax ID number, as well as other data.

Exercise 9-1

Preview a User Information Report on the screen by clicking on the User Information option, then choosing preview the report on the screen, then click on **Start**.

1. List some of the information included in the User Information Report.

_____

_____

_____

_____

Window Menu Options

The Window Menu option allows you to move quickly between the windows you have open. For example, if you open the Patient List, then choose a patient, you have two windows open. You can click back and forth between them by using this option and simply clicking on the window you wish to view. Each time you open a new window, that window will appear superimposed over the existing window. All windows remain open until you click on the icon in the upper-left corner and choose **Close** to close them, or until you click on their respective red X in the upper-right corner of each window.

This menu option also allows you to quickly close all the windows you have open by clicking on the Close All Windows option.

Help Menu Options

The Help Menu option provides you with information regarding the MediSoft system and how to use it. By clicking on this menu option, you can perform the following functions:

Bring up the **NDCMedisoft™ Help option**, which will tell you about any topic, how to access it, and/or how to perform the function (i.e., how to enter a new patient). The NDCMedisoft™ Help option can provide you with an easy reference tool if you forget how to accomplish a task in MediSoft.

It is also possible to print the information that you look up in the NDCMedisoft™ Help screen by looking up the information on the screen, then clicking on the **File** menu option in the upper-left corner, and choosing **Print Topic**.

The **Upgrades from NDCMediSoft™ for DOS** option provides instructions and tips for those people who have been using a DOS-based system and have files entered into the MediSoft for DOS system, which they wish to have copied into the MediSoft for Windows system. Converting these files from DOS to Windows can save tremendous amounts of time because each patient and their history (previous transactions) will not have to be reentered.

The **NDCMediSoft™ on the Web** option is a link to various Internet pages containing pertinent information regarding the MediSoft software.

The **Online Updates** option is a way to search the NDCMedisoft™ website for free updates for whatever program you are using.

The **Show Hints** option is an on/off key. If you wish MediSoft to provide you with hints on how to complete many of the fields in the MediSoft screen, click on this option. A check by the option means the hints will be shown. No check means the hints will not be shown.

The **Show Shortcut Keys** tells the MediSoft program whether or not you would like to see the shortcut keys to perform a function (usually Alt combined with a letter). A check by the option means the shortcut keys will be shown. No check means the shortcut keys will not be shown.

Each MediSoft program must be registered within 90 days of activation or the purchaser will be locked out of the program. The **Register Program** option provides you with the registration form, which must be completed to register your program.

The **About NDCMediSoft™** option provides you with the version number of the MediSoft program you are currently working in and whether it is a single-user version or one designed to be networked.

CHAPTER REVIEW

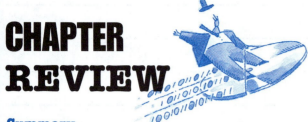

Summary

- The Edit Menu option deals primarily with the handling of text, often in specific windows. By using your mouse to highlight a portion of the text, you may choose to cut, copy, paste, or delete a portion of text.

- The Tools Menu option allows you to look up information regarding your system and its setup, as well as to use an on-screen calculator.
- The Windows Menu option allows you to move quickly between the windows you have open. It also allows you to quickly close all the windows you have open by clicking on the Close All Windows option.
- The Help Menu option provides you with information regarding the MediSoft system and how to use it.

Questions for Review

Directions: Answer the following questions without looking back into the material just covered. Write your answers in the space provided.

1. What four options are available in the Edit Menu?

  1. _____

  2. _____

  3. _____

  4. _____

2. What does the Tools Menu option allow you to do?

  _____

  _____

  _____

3. What is the purpose of the View File option?

  _____

  _____

4. How do you access the MediSoft calculator?

  _____

  _____

5. List the five options available under the Window Menu options.

  1. _____

2. _____

3. _____

4. _____

5. _____

If you were unable to answer any of the questions, refer back to that section, and then fill in the answers

10
Office Hours Menu Options

After completion of this chapter
you will be able to:

- Access the Office Hours Main Menu options.
- Set recurring appointments and breaks.
- Change the program options and create a customized appointment list.

Choosing the Appointment Book option under the Patient Management sidebar opens the Office Hours program. Office Hours is a separate scheduling and time management program. This program makes scheduling appointments simple and easy with just the use of a few keystrokes allowing you to enter, change, and delete patient appointments. You may also enter the Office Hours program through the main windows screen by choosing the Office Hours icon rather than the MediSoft program icon.

Menu options for the Office Hours program allow you to perform all necessary functions for setting up and tracking patient appointments.

Office Hours Main Menu Options

As with the MediSoft program, several main menu options occur across the top of the screen. Clicking on a main menu option will bring up a list of submenu options that you may choose from. The **Office Hours** program contains seven main menu options (**see Figure 10–1**):

1. File
2. Edit
3. View
4. Lists
5. Reports
6. Tools
7. Help

The **File Menu (see Figure 10–2)** option allows you to perform the following functions:

1. Open Practice
2. New Practice
3. Program Options
4. File Maintenance
5. Backup Data
6. Restore Data
7. Security Setup
8. Exit

The **Edit Menu (see Figure 10–3)** option allows you to perform what functions?

1. _____
2. _____
3. _____
4. _____
5. _____
6. _____
7. _____
8. _____

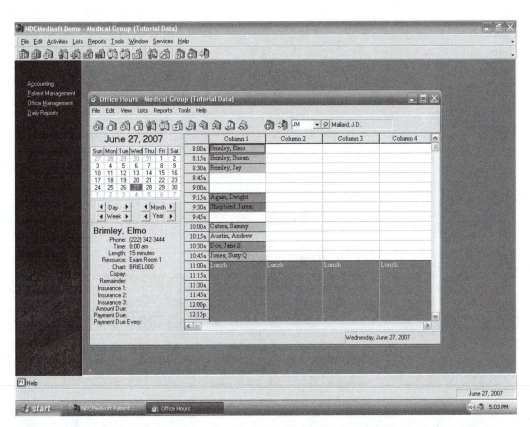

■ **Figure 10–1** Main Menu

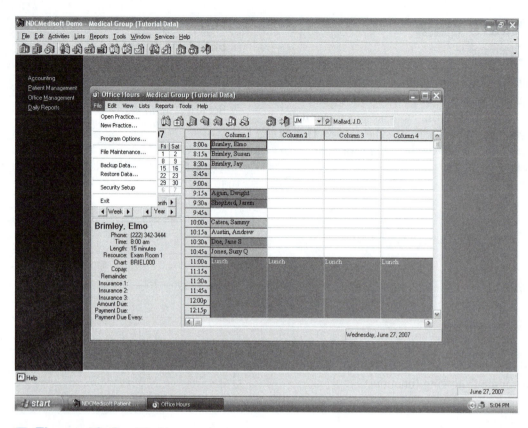

■ **Figure 10–2** File Menu

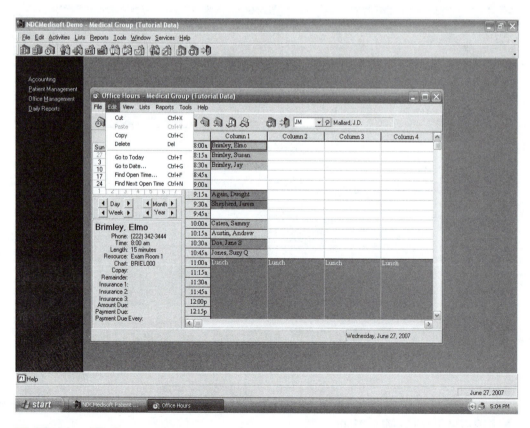

■ **Figure 10–3** Edit Menu

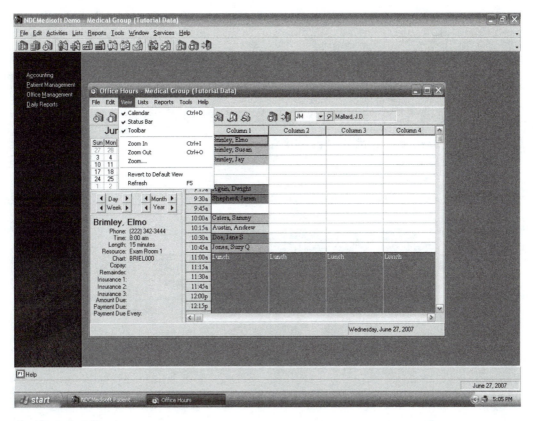

■ **Figure 10–4**   View Menu

The **View Menu (see Figure 10–4)** option allows you to perform what functions?

1. _____

2. _____

3. _____

4. _____

5. _____

6. _____

7. _____

8. _____

The **Lists Menu (see Figure 10–5)** option allows you to perform what functions?

1. _____

2. _____

3. _____

4. _____

5. _____

6. _____

The **Reports Menu (see Figure 10–6)** option allows you to perform what functions?

1. _____

2. _____

   A. _____

3. _____

4. _____

5. _____

6. _____

7. _____

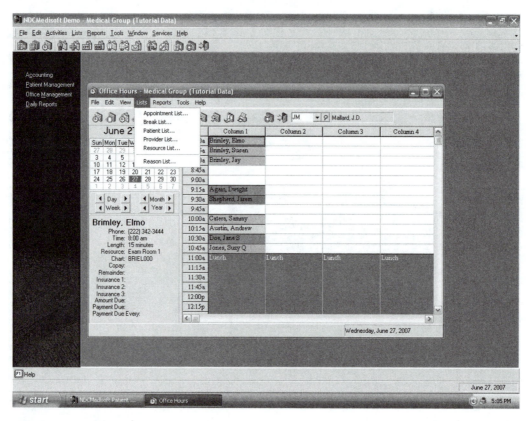

■ **Figure 10–5** Lists Menu

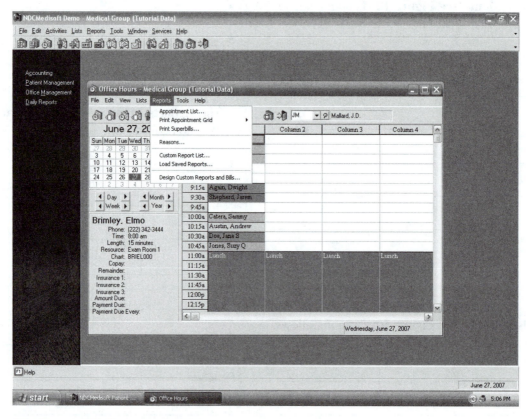

■ **Figure 10–6** Reports Menu

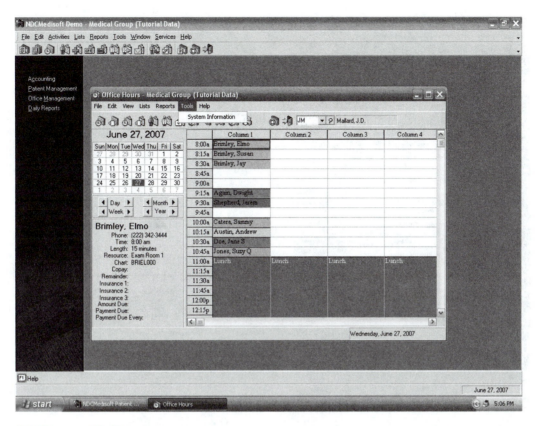

■ **Figure 10–7**   Tools Menu

The **Tools Menu (see Figure 10–7)** option allows you to perform what function?

1. _____

The **Help Menu (see Figure 10–8)** option allows you to perform what functions?

1. _____

2. _____

3. _____

4. _____

   A. _____

   B. _____

   C. _____

   D. _____

   E. _____

5. _____

File Menu Options

The File Menu option is the first main menu option, and it allows you to perform the following functions:

1. Open Practice
2. New Practice
3. Program Options
4. File Maintenance
5. Backup Data
6. Restore Data
7. Security Setup
8. Exit

Open Practice

This option allows you to open (retrieve) the data that has been stored regarding this practice. This includes data both about the practice and about the individual appointments that have been set up for that practice.

New Practice

This option allows you to create a new set of data for setting up appointments. If you have set up your practice

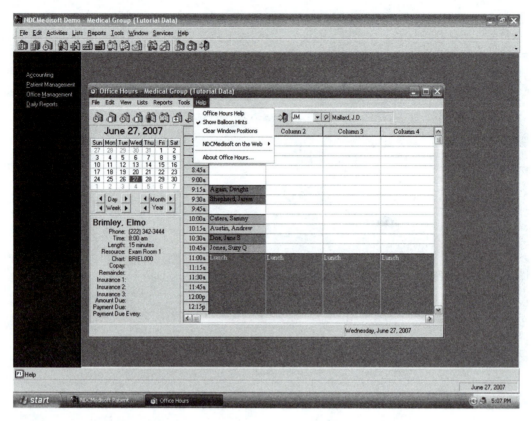

using the MediSoft program File Menu, that data will already have been created, and you will not need to create a new set of data.

If you have not previously set up data, enter the name of the doctor or practice, and then enter the data path where you would like this information to be stored.

Program Options

The program options file menu allows you to customize the appointment lists and reports in these ways:

1. The starting and ending time for the practice.
2. The number of minutes between each listed time (i.e., every half hour instead of every 15 minutes).
3. The number of booking columns (if your office has several treatment rooms).
4. Default Colors for Appointments, Scheduling Conflicts, and Breaks.

You can also specify whether you want the following options enabled or disabled:

1. Use Enter to move between fields.
2. Use automatic word capitalization.

3. Automatic Refresh.
4. Show notes on new appointment.

File Maintenance

Here you have the same File Maintenance options that appear in the MediSoft File Maintenance menu. However, these apply only to the data that has been entered into the Office Hours program (i.e., Appointment Lists, Patient Lists, and Provider Lists.) You may choose to rebuild these lists, pack them, back up data, purge data, or restore data. For additional information, see the File Maintenance options in Chapter 4.

Exit

This option allows you to exit the Office Hours program. If you entered the Office Hours program through the MediSoft Activities menu option, you will be returned to the MediSoft program.

Edit Menu Options

The Edit Menu option allows you to perform the following functions:

1. Cut
2. Paste

3. Copy
4. Delete
5. Go to Today
6. Go to Date
7. Find Open Time
8. Find Next Open Time

This allows you to cut, copy, paste, delete, and find appointments.

Cut allows you to cut an appointment. This is most often done when you wish to move an appointment from one time to another or from one date to another. The Cut and Paste functions remove the entry from its original location and post it to a new destination, resulting in one entry being made. To move an appointment, you would first highlight it, and then click on **Cut.** You would then use the mouse to move the cursor to where you wish to insert the appointment by changing the date (if necessary), and then use the Paste option to insert the information.

Copy allows you to copy an appointment. The Copy and Paste functions leave the entry in its original location and also post a copy of it to a new destination, resulting in two entries being made. First highlight the appointment you wish to copy. Then click on the **Copy** option. Then move your cursor to the position where you wish the appointment to be copied, and use the Paste option. This option is most often used when a patient is setting up two or more appointments. Using this option prevents you from having to reenter the patient information each time.

Paste allows you to insert the appointment that was last cut or copied into the current position of the cursor. It is used with Cut to move an appointment from one place to another or with Copy to make more than one appointment for the same patient.

Delete allows you to quickly delete an appointment. By clicking on this option, the highlighted appointment will be erased.

Using these options allows you to modify your appointment schedules faster than if you were to use the delete keys and/or type in the information again.

Go To Today allows you to quickly see appointments entered for today.

The **Go To Date** menu option allows you to quickly move from one date to another. After clicking on this option, you may choose to go to a specific date if it is known. There are also options for going to a date that is a specified number of days, weeks, months, or years from the current year. This is used when the provider requests that the patient return in a specified

period of time (i.e., two weeks) for a follow-up appointment. The years option is seldom used; however, providers who treat cancer patients may mark a date five years from the date the cancer is in remission (a patient may be considered cured if cancer free for five years), or patients can easily be scheduled for a yearly checkup using this option.

The **Find Open Time** option searches for available time slots in a provider's schedule. Fill in the length of the appointment and its start and end time then click on the day of the week you wish to schedule an appointment for and click **Search,** The program will display the time slot and show you if anything has been scheduled for that time and day.

The **Find Next Open Time** option allows you to search again if the first date was unacceptable for any reason.

View Menu Options

The view menu option allows you to indicate whether or not you would like the **calendar**, **status bar**, and/or **tool bar** to appear on the screen. A checkmark beside each option indicates it is viewable on the screen. No checkmark indicates it is not.

You can also **Zoom in** or **Zoom out** on the screen.

The **Refresh** option redraws the information on your screen so it appears properly. Otherwise data on the screen may seem to overlap.

Lists Menu Options

The Lists Menu option has six submenu options:

1. Appointment List
2. Break List
3. Patient List
4. Provider List
5. Resource List
6. Reason List

The Office Hours program automatically pulls the information in these lists from the Patients/Guarantors List and Providers List in the MediSoft program. These options allow you to edit or add patients, guarantors, providers, and staff members to the existing lists. The information that is added or changed here will also appear in the corresponding MediSoft list. The data that is entered here is the same as was entered in the MediSoft program. If you need further information on completing these fields, see Chapters 5 and 6.

Here you also have the opportunity to create lists of breaks, resources, and reasons. Breaks are items such as lunch or coffee breaks that may need to be scheduled into a provider's day. Resources are the rooms available for use (i.e., two exam rooms, a conference room, lunch room). Reasons are the reason a patient may be requesting an appointment or the type of patient they are (i.e., Medicare patient).

Reports Menu Options

The reports menu options allow you to print reports. The choices in this menu option include the following:

Appointment List: This option prints a list of appointments that have been scheduled.

Print Appointment Grid: This prints a list of appointments in grid format.

Print Superbills: This feature allows you to print superbills for patients. Superbills allow providers to quickly report the services performed and their diagnoses.

Reasons: Is a list of the reasons that have been entered into the computer.

Custom Report List: Is a list of all the custom reports that have been created by the practice.

Load Saved Reports: Allows you to load reports you may have previously saved.

Design Custom Reports and Bills: Allows you to create a report that has just what you want in it.

Once you have chosen any of these reports, you will be asked whether you want the report printed to the screen, to a file, or to the printer. If you choose to send the report to the screen you will still have the option of printing it after you view it.

Once you have chosen where the report will be sent, a new screen will allow you to choose the parameters. This is most often the date, provider, or chart (patient).

Tools Menu Options

The Tools Menu option contains the **System Information.** This option will bring up information about your system, including which version of Windows and DOS you are using, how much space you have available in your computer, and the type of printer you are using. This screen is for informational purposes only.

Help Menu Options

The Help Menu option provides you with information about the MediSoft system and how to use it. By clicking on this menu option, you can perform the following functions:

Bring up the **Office Hours Help** option, and it will tell you about any topic, how to access it, and/or how to perform the function (i.e., how to enter a new patient). The Office Hours Help option can provide you with an easy reference tool if you forget how to accomplish a task in MediSoft.

It is also possible to print the information that you look up in the Office Hours Help option and How to Use Help screens by looking up the information on the screen, then clicking on the File Menu option in the upper-left-hand corner, and choosing Print Topic.

The **Show Balloon Hints** option allows you to turn on and off the balloon hints that appear next to a field in which the cursor is placed. A checkmark beside this option indicates that the balloon hints will show. Clicking on this option will remove the checkmark, and the balloon hints will not show. The hints will still appear at the bottom of the page, regardless of whether this option is turned on or off.

Clear Window Positions allows you to take off the window options quickly.

The **NDCMediSoft™ on the Web** option allows you to immediately connect to the NDCMediSoft™ website. This item is simply an Internet link to their site.

The **Online Updates** option allows you to quickly receive online updates to the software. This is also a link to their website. It should be noted that in order for these options to work, your computer must have Internet access.

Finally, the **About Office Hours** option allows you to view which version of MediSoft you are using.

Search Options

This option is not found in all versions of MediSoft. However, this option allows you to search for information using many variables.

Quick Select Icons

Across the top of the screen are 14 quick select icons. These icons allow you to choose a function to perform without going through the process of selecting a menu option, then selecting a suboption. The quick select icons include the following:

1. Appointment Entry

 2. Break Entry

 3. Appointment List

 4. Break List

 5. Patient List

 6. Provider List

 7. Resource List

 8. Go To Date

 9. Search For Open Time Slot

 10. Search Again

 11. Go To Today

 12. Print Appointment List

 13. Help

 14. Exit

Let's look at each of these in a bit more depth.

Appointment Entry

This option opens a screen for entering information for a new appointment. This will be discussed in more detail in the next chapter.

Break Entry

This option allows you to create breaks in a provider's schedule. These can be either a single break or a recurring daily break in a provider's schedule (i.e., lunch from 12 p.m. to 1 p.m.). On some versions of Medi-Soft, this function was performed by two buttons, a Break Entry and a Recurring Break Entry option.

Appointment List

This option allows you to find an appointment quickly and easily when you do not have all the information on the appointment (i.e., date and time). For example, you can locate a patient's appointment by typing their name into the search field.

To find an appointment, click on this option. When the search window pops up, first choose the data you wish to sort by. Click on the **Search by** field, and choose whether you wish to search for an appointment by the chart number, the date of the appointment, the name of the patient, or the provider. Most often it will be easiest to search by the name of the patient. Once you have completed this field, click on the **Search for** field and begin entering the chart number, date of appointment, name of the patient, or the provider. You may enter all or part of the data. When you have entered data into this field, press enter. Any items that match the chart number, date, name, or provider will appear in the search window. The date and time of the

appointment will also appear to assist you in choosing the one you wish to see. Click on the item you wish to see, and the information will appear on the screen. If there is only one appointment that matches the information you have entered in the Search for field, that information will appear on the screen without the use of the search window.

Break List

This option displays a list of all scheduled breaks. This allows you to see when a provider is out of the office.

Patient List

This option shows you a list of the patients currently entered into the system and allows you to edit them. You may also add a new patient using this option. For more information, see the List menu option: Patients/Guarantors.

Provider List

This option shows you a list of the providers currently entered into the system and allows you to edit them. You may also add a new provider using this option.

Resource List

This is a list of the rooms that are available. Thus, if a provider has more than one exam room, an overlapping appointment can be scheduled in the second exam room.

Go To Date

This option allows you to quickly go to a specific date. For more information, see the Edit menu option Go To Date.

Search for Open Time Slot

This allows you to search for time slots that may be open on a specific date or at a specific time.

This can be especially helpful when you are setting up an appointment and the patient is looking for the earliest time the provider can see him or her.

To find available appointment times, click on the **Find** menu option. Enter the length of the appointment that the patient desires or will need. If you are unsure of the amount of time a certain procedure will take, look up the procedure using the appointment scheduling screen in the main menu. Entering a procedure number will allow the length of the appointment to show in the length field directly below the procedure.

Enter the beginning hour and minutes that the patient would consider coming in, then click on A.M. or P.M. to indicate morning or afternoon.

Enter the ending hour and minutes after which the patient is unable to come in, and then click on A.M. or P.M. to indicate morning or afternoon. Be sure there is an X next to any days that the patient would consider coming in for the appointment. The Office Hours program automatically enters an X on every day. Therefore, if the patient or the provider would rather not show up on any given day, click on that day, and the X will disappear. This is an on/off button, so clicking again will make the X reappear.

Once you have entered the data, click on the word **Search.** The program will automatically find the first available appointment date that meets the criteria that you have entered. If this date is unacceptable for any reason, choose the Search Menu option, and then click on **Search Again.** The program will then go to the next available appointment that meets your criteria.

Search Again

This option allows you to change the parameters and search a second or subsequent time.

Go to Today

Clicking on this icon returns the calendar to the current date.

Print Appointment List

This option prints a copy of the current appointment schedule that is shown on the screen.

Help

This option will allow you to access the help screen.

Exit

This option allows you to exit the Office Hours program. If you entered the Office Hours program through the MediSoft Activities menu option, you will be returned to the MediSoft program.

Be sure to save your work before you exit the Office Hour program.

Show/Hide Hints

This is an on/off function key that commands the program to either show or hide the hints that appear in a balloon near the icon or field that the cursor is in.

CHAPTER REVIEW

Summary

- The Appointment Book option opens the Office Hours program. This is a separate MediSoft program that allows you to enter, change, and delete patient appointments. The Office Hours program can also be accessed through the main windows screen by choosing the Office Hours icon.

- The File Menu option allows you to open a practice, create a practice, back up and restore data, change program options, perform file maintenance, and exit the program.
- The Edit Menu options allow you to cut, copy, paste, or delete an appointment that was entered. The Go To Date menu option allows you to quickly move from one date to another.
- The View, Lists, Reports, Tools, and Help Menu options allow you to select screen display options, retrieve patient and provider information that has been stored, look at the system information for the program you are using, print reports, and ask for help in completing a field or using an option.

Questions for Review

Directions: Answer the following questions without looking back into the material just covered. Write your answers in the space provided.

1. What menu option allows you to cut and paste data?

   _____

   _____

   _____

2. What menu option allows you to zoom in and out on the screen?

   _____

   _____

   _____

3. What menu option allows you to print out an appointment list?

   _____

   _____

   _____

4. What menu option do you use to find an open time slot?

   _____

   _____

5. What is the purpose of the Break Entry icon?

   _____

   _____

   _____

   If you were unable to answer any of the questions, refer back to that section, and then fill in the answers.

11

Appointment Book

After completion of this chapter
you will be able to:

- Set an appointment for a patient.
- Identify and use the quick select icons.

In this chapter we will discuss the Office Hours main screen, the changing of dates and providers, and the entering of appointments.

The Main Screen

The main screen is used for entering appointments on a provider's schedule. Before setting up an appointment, it is important to ensure that you are working on the appointment calendar for the correct provider and are also working on the correct date.

Choosing a Provider

The first step in setting up an appointment is to choose the correct provider. Each provider has their own appointment calendar. You choose the provider you wish to work on by clicking on the Provider Field in the upper-right corner of the screen. This will bring up a list of all the providers who are currently entered into the system. For a provider to have an appointment calendar set up, they must have previously been entered into the Provider List screen in either the MediSoft program, or in the Office Hours program (see Provider List for further information).

Choosing a Date

The Office Hours program shows only one date at a time on the screen. To properly set appointments,

breaks, meetings, or any other items into a provider's schedule, you must be sure that the correct date is showing on the screen.

The Office Hours program will automatically bring up the current date on the screen. To change the date, use the arrows below the calendar on the left of the screen to select the correct date. This will bring up a calendar of the month and year you have chosen. The calendar will show each date on the appropriate day of the month for that month and year. To choose a date, simply click on the date.

Once you have completed these steps, the appointment calendar for the chosen provider on the chosen date will appear on the right half of the screen.

Setting Up an Appointment

Setting up an appointment is the most commonly performed function in the Office Hours program.

To set up an appointment for a patient, first be sure you have chosen the correct date and the correct provider. Then double-click on the time you wish to set up an appointment. The Appointment Entry screen will appear. Enter the following information in each of the appointment screen fields:

Exercise 11-1

Enter an appointment for Candy Dunnitt on 1/19/CCYY at 1:30 p.m. with Dr. Phil Goode. She will be having a straightforward office visit and glucose check to monitor her diabetes. Add the message that the patient's weight should be checked during the visit.

Chart/Name: Enter the chart number of the patient. As soon as you begin typing a chart number or name, the automatic search feature will bring up a list of all patients whose chart number matches the letters you have typed. At this point you may click on one of these numbers or names, or continue typing in the complete chart number. You may also use the arrow down to bring up a list of all patients or the magnifying glass to perform a search for a patient.

Phone: If the patient's phone number was previously entered into the Patient List, it will automatically appear here. If the number is not correct or if the patient can be more easily reached at a different number, enter that number here.

Resource: Enter the location where the appointment will take place. This field has a search option.

Note: Enter any message you wish printed on the appointment list in the space next to the patient's appointment. This can be a reminder for the provider to check the patient's weight or blood pressure, or something more personal such as asking about a family member (i.e., son Bob has cancer). As you type, some characters will scroll off the left side of the field, but they will still print on the appointment list.

Case: If there is more than one case associated with this patient, choose the appropriate case for this visit.

Reason: Enter the reason the patient is requesting the appointment.

Length: Enter the number of minutes the procedure is expected to take. If the procedure takes longer than a single space (usually 15 minutes in length), then the Office Hours program will place the patient's name in the time slot for the first 15 minutes and will shade out the remaining number of minutes to indicate that this time is taken by the above patient. Shading is done in 15-minute intervals. Therefore, if you have a patient with a 40-minute appointment, the patient's name will be shown in the first 15-minute time slot, and the following time slot only will be shaded. If the appointment is for 45 minutes, two additional time slots will be shaded. Because of this, it is important to schedule patients in 15-minute intervals. If you wish to change the amount of time in each appointment interval, use the File menu option, click on Program Options and alter the interval (see File Menu options for additional information).

Date: Enter the desired date of the appointment.

Time: Enter the time of the appointment.

Provider: Enter the name of the provider who will be seeing the patient for this appointment.

Repeat: This option allows you to set up multiple appointments at a single time. For example, if a woman is pregnant, she may need to see the doctor every month. If she would like an appointment on the 5th of every month at the same time, the repeat option can be used to choose a monthly appointment time. Repeat options include daily, weekly, monthly, and yearly options. Repeat appointments may also be used to block out a provider's schedule. For example, if the provider has a meeting at the same time every week, this function can block out that time every week.

Change: Clicking this button allows you to set up and/or change the frequency of the repeat appointments.

Procedure Code: Enter the procedure code for the service that the provider will be performing. This code should previously have been entered in the Procedure Code List in MediSoft. If not, you will need to add it there before entering it here. You may also use the arrow down to bring up a list of all procedure codes or the magnifying glass to perform a search for a procedure code. If a time was included when the procedure code was entered, the appropriate amount of time would be scheduled for the visit.

After you have completed the preceding fields, clicking **Save** will place the appointment into the appointment calendar and save the information.

CHAPTER REVIEW

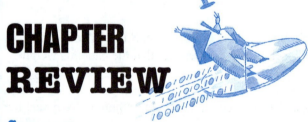

Summary

- You have now completed the tutorial part of the MediSoft Training Program. You should now have a good working knowledge of the MediSoft Patient Billing software program. However, many things take practice to learn. The following Simulated Work portion of the training program will give you practice entering information in the previously mentioned screens, running reports, and performing all the necessary tasks of a medical billing specialist.

- You will have the opportunity to enter numerous patients, as well as claims, payments, appointments, and other activities. By the end of the Simulated Work Program, you should be proficient not only in the use of the MediSoft Patient Accounting Program, but also in many of the daily tasks of medical billing.

Questions for Review

Directions: Answer the following questions without looking back into the material just covered. Write your answers in the space provided.

1. Before you enter an appointment, be sure you have chosen the correct _____

_____ and _____.

2. How do you choose the time you wish to set up an appointment?

_____

_____

_____

3. What is the purpose of the Resource field?

_____

_____

_____

4. What information is entered in the Reason field?

_____

_____

_____

5. What is the purpose of the Repeat field?

_____

_____

_____

If you were unable to answer any of the questions, refer back to that section, and then fill in the answers.

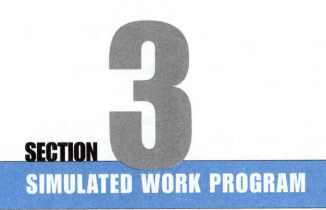

SECTION 3
SIMULATED WORK PROGRAM

SIMULATED WORK PROGRAM

ENTERING A CLAIM "INTO THE SYSTEM"

JANUARY 14, CCYY

JANUARY 21, CCYY

FEBRUARY 4, CCYY

MARCH 4, CCYY

Simulated Work Program

Congratulations on making it through the tutorial portion. Now you are ready to step into the shoes of a real medical biller and enter a simulated work program.

As a medical biller, it is your job to enter new patients into the system (computerized or manual), bill for services rendered, and keep an accurate log of the provider's accounts. Often you will be required to enter a new doctor or patient into the system. Other times the doctor or patient will already be in the system, and you must locate his or her existing records.

In an actual office setting, doctors will submit numerous patient charge slips, usually one for each patient seen. A doctor can see 20 to 30 patients in an average day, which means creating 20 to 30 patient billings and updating their charts every day. Add in phone calls, dealing with patients, handling mail, receiving payments, and rebilling secondary insurance or patients for any balances left, and you can see how busy the job can become.

This simulated work program is set up to give you practical knowledge in the day-to-day activities of the medical biller. It simulates many of the duties you will be asked to perform in an office setting. Additionally, you will have the opportunity to code and bill numerous types of claims, including physician's services, lab, surgery, assistant surgery, anesthesia, durable medical equipment, and ambulance claims. During this simulated work program, be sure to use the dates indicated in the text. **In each case the year CCYY or YY should be replaced with the current year. The year PY should be replaced with the prior year (i.e., if you are completing this in 2006, CCYY = 2006 and PY = 2005).**

Note Regarding Dates:

Please note that when YY is used in reference to a date, the YY indicates the current year (12/01/YY). When PY is used in reference to a date, the PY indicates the prior year or last year (12/01/PY). When NY is used in reference to a date, NY indicates the next year (12/01/NY).

Note Regarding Birth Dates:

Birth dates will be referenced with CCYY − ## (where the ## is the age of the patient). This indicates to subtract the ## from the current year to determine the birth year.

Example: What is the birth date 10/04/CCYY − 14, if CCYY = 2006?

2006 − 14 = 1992, therefore the birth date = **10/04/1992**

Feel free to use other available resources to complete the assignments. On the job you will often have many of these resources available to you. These can include CPTs®, ICD-9-CMs, medical dictionaries, medical terminology books, medical billing instruction books, and reference books on completing forms. If you have difficulty remembering how to complete a screen, do not hesitate to consult the manual that describes the data entry.

In a normal office, only one or perhaps two people in a family will seek treatment. Then an extended period of time elapses before treatment is again sought (unless a chronic condition exists). We have compressed several visits into a three-month period to allow you to gain experience compiling charts, figuring deductibles paid, and seeing how one claim may affect others in a family group. As such, the simulated work program covers five days, which are spread throughout this three-month period. When beginning a new day's work, be sure to change the computer to the correct date, otherwise, data may be posted incorrectly or appear incorrectly on day sheets and other reports.

Additionally, we have limited the scenarios to 14 families so you do not have to enter an excessive number of providers or unrelated patients.

To save paper and printing costs, we have summarized the information contained on charge slips rather than presenting the entire charge slip. Likewise, we have included information on dependents on the same form as the insured. This prevents duplication of items such as address, phone number, and insurance plan information.

Go through the exercises step by step. Do not skip any or move on until you have fully completed a step. Otherwise your totals on subsequent exercises may be incorrect. The exception to this is for those who have completed the tutorial portion in section 2 of this text. You may skip items 3–7 because they were done at that time.

If you are unsure how to complete a step, refer back to the information contained in the tutorial portion. Some steps will ask you to enter data, create reports, or deal with individuals on the telephone. Most steps will deal directly with data contained in this text; however, it is assumed that you will have previously received training on the basic functions of medical billing (i.e., dealing with patients, record keeping, CPT® and ICD-9-CM coding, completing claim forms, privacy issues, and medical charting). You will need to rely on this knowledge to complete some exercises.

At the end of each day's steps is a section for recording additional information or other data or confirmation that may be needed. If additional information is needed from a patient or other party, list it here and then complete a "Request for Additional Information" form, which can be found in the back of the book. The outside margins in this section are wider to allow for note taking, and the exercises are marked with an Item checkoff box to help keep track of where you stopped working.

You will also encounter a number of critical thinking exercises. These exercises present you with a situation and ask what you would do. They are intended to help you make the transition from trainee to medical biller. Each situation involves a scenario that you may or may not have had training in or experienced before. Be sure to take time to think about your answer. Often there are pitfalls in a situation that may not be obvious. You should call on the previous learning you have had in this field and remember all rules and regulations regarding privacy issues, collections, and all other aspects of the job.

Here you will have the time to think through an answer, whereas on the job you may not. Try to place yourself in the situation and respond appropriately. Read through the scenario and then write your response in the space provided.

Critical thinking exercises generally do not affect the data entry for the other assignments. If you are unable to come up with the correct answer, do not worry about it. It will not critically affect subsequent entries. Just make your best guess. At the end of the simulated work program, ask the instructor for the answer to those items with which you had difficulty.

If it is easy for you to respond with the correct answer, Great! You have learned how to deal with that situation. If you find that your response has faults, do not worry. These situations will probably be the ones that you remember the most. If so, you will have achieved the purpose of this book and learned from the experience of being a medical biller. Hopefully, this book will give you the practical experience both to apply the training you have had and to think on your feet when presented with a new and unusual situation.

If you are completely stumped, there are clues listed for many of the critical thinking exercises at the back of this section. You should attempt to answer the question on your own, then look up the clue. It may provide you with confirmation of your answer or provide you with additional information for handling the situation.

Manual and Computerized Entry Instructions

This simulated work program may be used by students who are using a manual or pegboard system, as well as those using any computerized medical billing program.

Specific instructions for completing data manually are indicated with the ☐ symbol. Specific instructions for completing data on a computerized system 🖥 are indicated by the symbol. Use only those instructions that are appropriate for your system. Instructions that are appropriate for all users are not indented behind a symbol.

For example: All students or trainees using the simulated work program should read and utilize data that appears in this format.

☐ Only those students or trainees using a manual or pegboard system should use these specific instructions.

🖥 Only those students or trainees using a computerized medical billing system should use these specific instructions.

Entering a Claim "Into the System"

At various times patients will need to be billed for services rendered. On the job the provider will complete a superbill or charge slip for the patient that shows the services performed and the related diagnoses. To save paper, the simulated work program will list all the pertinent information regarding services performed in a brief scenario paragraph. This paragraph will be headed with a **CLAIM NUMBER**. To help keep track of papers for this course, place the appropriate claim number in the upper-right-hand corner of each 1500 Health Insurance Claim Form created.

To give you practice in coding procedures and diagnoses, the appropriate CPT® and ICD-9-CM codes have not been listed. To complete the billing on a claim, use the CPT® and ICD-9-CM books to code the procedure and diagnoses. Unless otherwise indicated, all office visits should be considered established patients.

To "enter a claim into the system" means to complete each of the following steps.

   a. Complete a 1500 form for the patient visit. If you are not using two-part 1500 forms, write up two forms or make a copy of the 1500 when it is completed. One copy will go in the patient chart, and the other will be mailed to the insurance carrier.

   b. Update the patient's chart, including patient ledger cards and patient statements.

   c. If the patient made a payment, create a receipt.

   a. If you have not previously done so, enter the patient and any other family members into the Patient Information database.

   b. Enter the CPT® codes into the Procedure Information screens. Some procedures may have been previously entered using Document 4. If so, these procedures do not need to be reentered. If a procedure has already been entered, the data will appear on the screen when you enter the code into the Procedure Code field.

   c. Enter the ICD-9-CM codes into the Diagnosis Code Information screen. Some diagnoses may have been previously entered using Document 5. If so, these diagnoses do not need to be reentered. If a diagnosis has already been entered, the data will appear on the screen when you enter the code into the Diagnosis Code field.

   d. Enter the charges as shown on the claim scenarios. If a payment was made, enter the payment and print a walkout receipt before saving the data.

Many computer systems allow you to print out all patient claims that were entered in a single day. For this reason there will be a notation at the end of each day for computerized billing users to print out the 1500 forms that they have entered for that day. Using two-part 1500 forms is suggested. If you are using one-part forms, print out two copies or make a photocopy of the form after it is completed. One copy of the form will go in the patient file, and the second copy will be mailed to the insurance carrier for payment.

Getting Started

You are now ready to start the simulated work program. If you are using computerized billing software, you should first become familiar with it. You need not become proficient as you will get plenty of practice using the program during this portion of the text. However, you should be familiar with how the program operates and the correct screen for entering various pieces of data.

When entering transactions (charges or payments), be sure to tie the payment(s) to the proper charge(s). Doing this allows you to keep track of the amount that has been paid on each visit.

JANUARY 14, CCYY

1   Today's date is January 14, CCYY. Change the date in the computer to January 14, CCYY.

2   Count petty cash. How much is in the cash envelope? _____

3   At the beginning of each year, your office sends out a patient information sheet to each patient and asks them to complete and return it. This allows the office to keep their information current and ensures that any changes are updated at least yearly. Two more patient information sheets arrive over the fax machine (Documents 5 & 6). Review the patient information sheets and create charts for each family and patient. Enter the data from the patient information sheets into the computer. (NOTE: CHS attempts to get a picture of each patient and their family. However, if not all members of the family are treated by the practice, only the information for those members being treated will be included on the Patient Information Sheet).

4   You receive another sheet showing additional doctors in the CHS family (Document 7). Add the new doctors to the Provider Information database.

5 Sherry Attricks scuttles up to the window and begins tapping her fingers impatiently on the counter. Behind her, her grandson plops himself into a chair while holding his stomach. Mrs. Attricks hands you a patient information sheet (Document 8) and two charge slips. "I hope this won't take long," she exclaims. "I wasn't planning on scheduling *two* appointments today!" Create a patient and family chart then enter these charges into the system.

CLAIM 1
The claim for Ox O'Gen was processed in the Activities Menu chapter.

CLAIM 2
Petey Attricks received a comprehensive, high complexity exam ($190) in Dr. Phil Goode's office on 1/14/YY. A blood sample was taken ($15). Diagnosis: Abdominal Pain, Gastroenteritis. Petey received an immediate referral to Dr. Ben Dover, Gastroenterologist.

CLAIM 3
Petey Attricks received a new patient comprehensive confirmatory consultation, of moderate complexity performed in the office ($275) by Dr. Ben Dover on 1/14/YY. Patient was referred by Dr. Phil Goode. Diagnosis: Gallstones.

6 Dr. Dover prefers to collect the estimated patient portion of the charges at the time of the visit. You call the insurance carrier and find out that Petey has a $125 deductible, and none of it has been paid. Insurance pays 80%. Estimate the patient's portion of the charges.

What are the total charges? _____

What is the estimated insurance payment? _____

What is the estimated patient portion? _____

Sherry makes a payment for the preceding amount with check #1930 (in the Window Payments section behind the documents). Fill in the correct amount on the check. Enter it into the system. Be sure to cut out the check and put it in your petty cash envelope.

7 Sherry Attricks also asks for an appointment for herself with Dr. Sickman. Set up an appointment on 1/22/YY at 3:30 p.m. The appointment will take approximately 30 minutes. Use Dr. Sickman's appointment calendar (Document 9). Enter the appointment into the computer.

8 Suddenly you look up and there is someone at the window. Codie Pendent smiles at the recognition and hands you the following charge slip information. "My daughter was hurrying to answer the door this morning and tripped and fell," she explains. Enter the charges.

CLAIM 4
Dee Pendent received a minimal service exam in Dr. Goode's office ($35) today. Diagnosis: Multiple Contusions and Abrasions.

9 Ima Knose arrives at the window after her visit with Dr. Goode. She hands you a patient information sheet (Document 10) and charge slips containing the following information. Create a patient and family chart. Enter these charges into the system.

CLAIM 5
Ima Knose received a minimal office visit ($40), two subcutaneous injections were given ($30 each), on 1/14/YY; supplies and materials: ($12). Diagnosis: Hypoestrogenism, Hyperlipidemia. A cash payment of $25 was made for this visit (see Window Payments section). Patient requests a receipt.

10 During the same visit Ron E. Knose also received treatment. Enter these charges.

CLAIM 6

Ron E. Knose received an expanded exam with history performed by Dr. Phil Goode in the office ($85) on 1/14/YY. Patient complained of pain in the ear and a sore throat. A diagnosis of otitis media and acute pharyngitis was determined. An intramuscular antibiotic injection was given ($30). Another intramuscular antibiotic injection for ($26) was given. Symptoms first appeared 12/29/PY. A cash payment of $20 was made for this visit. The patient needs a receipt.

11 Sue Pervisor, the office manager, has asked for a copy of your day sheets at the end of each day. Day sheets show all patients seen, procedures done, or payments received during a given day. Print each of the day sheets. Use 01/14/YY as the date of the report. The report should include all entries.

12 Print a transaction list. Use 01/14/YY as the date of the report. The report should include all entries. Check both of these reports. If there are any errors, correct them before proceeding.

13 Print a deposit slip listing each check by number. Attach all checks and cash payments to the deposit slip.

14 Reconcile petty cash. Count all money remaining in petty cash and be sure you have the same amount left at the end of the day as you started with at the beginning. If not, determine exactly where the missing amount is.

15 Print all the claims you have entered today. If you are using one-part forms, print two copies (see following exercise).

16 Prepare claims for mailing. Place one copy of the claim in the patient file. Place the second copy together with all claims for a single carrier. Print or write address labels and attach them to the claims. Place these in the folder for completed insurance claims.

17 Is any additional information or confirmation needed regarding today's transactions? If so, what is it and how would you go about getting it?

_____

_____

_____

_____

18 Stop and check that all assignments are correct before continuing on to the next date.

JANUARY 21, CCYY

19 Today's date is January 21, CCYY. Change the date in the computer to January 21, CCYY.

20 Count petty cash. How much is in the cash envelope? _____

21 You check the fax machine and find a patient information sheet (Document 11). Create a patient chart for this family. Enter the data from the patient information sheet into the computer.

22 You receive a letter from Rover Insurers, Inc. confirming that Codie Pendent has received preauthorization for 10 psychiatric treatments with Dr. Reed Mi. Mind, commencing on January 15, CCYY. The preauthorization number is 1839A1B, authorized by D. Carrier. Dx: Adjustment Disorder. Enter this information into the patient's record.

23 As a medical biller, you should be familiar with at least some of the terms of the contracts for your patients. This allows you to inform the doctor and patient of any contract provisions, which could provide greater insurance reimbursement. For example, some contracts pay 100% for preadmission testing. Informing the doctor and patient of this allows them to make an informed decision regarding treatment.

At your request, Blue Corporation, Red Enterprises, and White Corporation have sent you copies of their contracts (Documents 12–14). Complete an insurance coverage sheet for each family. Blank insurance coverage sheets are in the Forms section in the back of this book. The completed insurance coverage sheets should be filed in the family's file, behind the patient information sheet.

When completing the insurance coverage sheets, list the name of the insured and their dependents across the bottom of the sheet. Use any previous claims and insurance payments to estimate the amount of deductible and coinsurance paid. This information should be considered estimated until confirmed by a phone call to the insurance carrier. Be sure that the address and phone number information is correct, and complete in the Insurance Information screen on the computer. If incorrect or incomplete, update the information.

24 Cab N. Fever enters the office with his children, Scarlet and Ty Phoid. The family had been hiking in the woods this morning on Mount Mountain. Ty has asthma and had an asthmatic attack. He is having dyspnea, though not severe. His father would like him checked out. Mr. Fever fills out a patient information sheet (Document 15). He is unsure of the correct payment order for the insurances that cover his children. Determine the correct order of insurance, and then create family and patient charts. Also be sure to add the diagnosis of asthma to Ty's patient information sheet if it was not listed by his father. Enter the patient information into the computer.

25 D. Jobb Dunnitt steps out of the treatment room with his daughter V. Iris Dunnitt. He hands you a charge slip showing the following charges. Enter the charges into the system.

CLAIM 7
Dr. Sickman performed a problem-focused office visit ($55) on V. Iris. Diagnosis: Rhinovirus.

Mr. Dunnitt asks how much the patient's portion for the visit will be. You contact his insurance carrier and find that V. Iris has not yet paid any of her deductible. Using the information contained on the patient insurance coverage sheet, determine how much the deductible and estimated patient's portion of the bill will be.

What are the total charges? _____

What is the estimated insurance payment? _____

What is the estimated patient portion? _____

Mr. Dunnitt writes a check (#1805 in the Windows Payment Section) for the preceding amount and asks for a receipt. Fill in the amount on the patient's check. Return to the transaction screen, enter the payment, and print him a receipt.

26 Ty Phoid and Cab N. Fever step out of the office. Mr. Fever hands you a charge slip for the following charges.

CLAIM 8
Ty received an office visit, low complexity ($150). Diagnosis: Asthma, Dyspnea.

27 You find claim information on the following patient visit in your IN box. Enter these charges into the system.

CLAIM 9

Codie Pendent received individual psychotherapy performed by Dr. Reed Mi. Mind, Psychiatrist, in the office on 1/17/YY ($160). Individual psychological testing was administered for five hours on 1/17/YY ($575). Diagnosis: Adjustment Disorder.

28 Mr. Shay Kee Hart toddles up to the window with a new patient information sheet (Document 16). He has just been seen by Dr. Yu B. Sickman, and the following services were rendered. Make up a patient chart and enter the following charges into the system.

CLAIM 10

Office visit, established, high complexity ($190), Urinalysis ($30). Diagnosis: Lou Gehrig's Disease.

When you finish with the claim form, Mr. Hart announces, "I would like to pay for the estimated patient portion of the visit at this time, including my yearly deductible. Here's my check (#1796 from the Window Payments section). You can fill in the amount for me. I would also like something showing me how you came up with my amount and a receipt for it."

Create the information Mr. Hart wants, then complete the check and process the payment.

29 Take a moment to make sure all of your patient charts are up to date and are placed neatly in alphabetical order.

30 You check your IN box and find two charge slips. The following claim information was received from Dr. Yu B. Sickman. Enter these charges into the system.

CLAIM 11

Ron E. Knose received an expanded exam with low complexity in the office on 1/20/YY ($85). His symptoms first appeared on 12/29/PY. He had previously seen Dr. Goode, but his symptoms have not cleared. An injection of penicillin was given ($25). Also a throat culture was done ($20) and a Urine dip ($30). Diagnosis: Upper Respiratory Infection.

CLAIM 12

Carla Poole was brought into the office on 1/14/YY with a laceration of the left index finger. Mr. Poole stated that Carla's finger was run over by a skate on 1/8/YY. The finger appears to be infected. An expanded visit of low complexity was performed ($85). An x-ray of the finger was done ($40). A sterile tray was used ($50) to prep and wrap the finger.

31 The auditors have just finished checking last year's accounts. They needed more information for why adjustments were made to decide whether they can be allowed. The entire office spent numerous hours looking up the information in the patient records. To prevent this from happening again, Sue Pervisor has created additional procedure codes that further clarify why adjustments were made (Document 17). Enter these codes and descriptions into the Procedure Code Information screen. Be sure that when you abbreviate the description, all pertinent information is included.

32 Dr. Sickman's receptionist has set up a number of appointments in Dr. Sickman's calendar (Document 9). She asks you to add these to the computer and also schedule the following appointment in the doctor's appointment calendar.

Pat Prescott would like an appointment on 1/22/YY at 3 p.m. for 30 minutes.

33 Dr. Will Kutteroff calls and asks you to schedule outpatient surgery for Rhea Ality for excision of a pilonidal cyst on 2/1/YY from 2:30 p.m. to 4 p.m. at CHS Community Hospital. Place the information for the surgery in the doctor's appointment schedule.

34 Sherry Attricks steps up to the window with a charge slip. Enter these charges into the system.

CLAIM 13

Sherry Attricks had the following tests performed in the office on 1/21/YY by Dr. Yu B. Sickman. Basic Metabolic Panel ($80), sodium ($21), potassium ($21), cholesterol ($25), and calcium ($20). Diagnosis: Venous Insufficiency, Varicose Veins. The patient pays $45 for this visit by check #1932 (see Window Payments section). Ms. Attricks would like a receipt.

35 Print a set of day sheets.

36 Print or write up a deposit slip for all monies received. Attach all checks and cash payments to it.

37 Reconcile petty cash. Count all money remaining in petty cash and be sure you have the same amount left at the end of the day as you started with at the beginning. If not, determine exactly where the missing amount is.

38 Print all the claims you have entered today. If you are using one-part forms, print two copies (see following exercise).

39 Prepare claims for mailing. Place one copy of the claim in the patient file. Place the second copy together with all claims for a single carrier. Print or write address labels and attach them to the claims. Place these in the folder for completed insurance claims.

40 Is any additional information or confirmation needed for today's transactions? If so, what?

_____

_____

_____

_____

_____

_____

41 Stop and check that all assignments are correct before continuing on to the next date.

FEBRUARY 4, CCYY

42 Today's date is February 4, CCYY. Change the date in the computer to February 4, CCYY.

43 Count petty cash. How much is in the cash envelope? _____

44 Included in the mail is a detailing of charges paid by Winter Insurance, one of the insurance carriers (Document 18). Credit the appropriate amounts to the correct accounts, and then do any balance billing to either the patient or an additional insurance carrier. When billing a secondary insurance payer, be sure to attach a copy of the EOB. Data for other patients should be redacted (blacked out). A secondary copy of the EOB need not be attached when you are balance billing the patient. The insurance carrier should have already sent them a copy of the EOB.

45 Three envelopes contain patient checks (Document 19). Credit these payments to the proper accounts.

46 D. Jobb Dunnitt steps up to the window with a charge slip. Enter these charges into the system.

CLAIM 14
Candy Dunnitt was seen by Dr. Sickman today for diabetes mellitus. An expanded exam with history was performed ($85) in the office. A routine blood glucose strip was done ($40) to check the blood sugar.

47 Also included in the mail is a detailing of charges paid by Rover Insurers, Inc. and Ball Insurance Carriers, two of the insurance carriers (Documents 20 and 21). Credit the appropriate amounts to the correct accounts, and then do any balance billing to either the patient or an additional insurance carrier. When billing a secondary insurance payer, be sure to attach a copy of the EOB. Data for other patients should be redacted (sensitive or classified information from a document should be removed prior to its release). A copy of the EOB need not be attached when you are balance billing the patient. The insurance carrier should have already sent them a copy of the EOB.

48 The following claim information was received from Dr. Ben Dover, gastroenterologist. Enter these charges into the system.

CLAIM 15
Petey Attricks received a hospital admit of moderate complexity performed on 1/14/YY ($180). On 1/15/YY, Dr. Dover performed a cholecystectomy with exploration of common duct ($2,060), which includes follow-up hospital visits performed on 1/16/YY and 1/17/YY and a discharge performed on 1/18/YY. Diagnosis: Calculus Cholecystitis. Patient hospitalized 1/14/YY through 1/18/YY at CHS Community Hospital.

CLAIM 16
Office surgery was performed by Dr. Ben Dover on Andy Pendent for a diagnosis of hemorrhoids. An anoscopy ($130) was performed on 1/17/YY. A hemorrhoidectomy, external, complete ($550) was also performed on 1/17/YY. Proctosigmoidoscopy ($100) and removal of polyp ($75) were performed on 1/18/YY. Mr. Pendent made a cash payment of $50 on 1/18/YY (see Window Payments section).

49 Dr. Dover asks you to estimate the patient's portion of the preceding charges and send the patient a bill. For Petey Attricks:

You call the insurance carrier and find out that he has not satisfied any of his deductible. However, you had previously sent in a bill for this patient, which has probably not been paid by the insurance carrier yet. Use the insurance coverage sheet to determine his deductible. Estimate the patient's portion of the preceding charges.

What are the total charges? _____

What is the estimated insurance payment? _____

What is the estimated patient portion? _____

For Andy Pendent:

You call the insurance carrier and find out that Mr. Pendent has not satisfied any of his deductible. Use the insurance coverage sheet to determine his deductible. Estimate the patient's portion of the preceding charges.

What are the total charges? _____

What is the estimated insurance payment? _____

What is the estimated patient portion? _____

How much was paid by the patient? _____

How much does the patient still owe? _____

Write a letter to the responsible party for each of the preceding patients requesting payment of the estimated portion of the patient's bill. Be sure to indicate that if the insurance carrier does not cover the entire billed amount there may be additional charges owed by the patient.

50 The following claim information was received from Dr. Yu B. Sickman. Enter these charges into the system.

CLAIM 17

D. Jobb Dunnitt came into CHS Urgent Care Trauma Center complaining of difficulty breathing. A problem-focused exam with straightforward decision making was performed ($120) on 1/23/YY. Dr. Sickman ordered a complete blood count with manual differential ($25) and a CO_2 response curve ($80). Because the patient was diagnosed with chronic bronchitis, a chest x-ray with two views was performed ($60). The patient was also diagnosed with asbestosis. The first visit pertaining to this illness was on 1/9/YY. A payment of $60 was made for this visit by patient check #1809 (see Window Payments section). The patient requests a receipt.

Remember to add the diagnoses of Chronic Bronchitis and Asbestosis to the patient information sheet if they are not already indicated.

CLAIM 18

Dee Pendent was brought into the office on 1/22/YY by her mother. Mrs. Pendent stated that Dee tripped at home and hit her head on the cement driveway. She was treated for a bloody nose and complained of headache and neck stiffness. A detailed exam of moderate complexity was performed ($130). A complete x-ray of the skull was taken ($85). Also a complete x-ray of the cervical spine was done ($100).

CLAIM 19

D. Jobb Dunnitt was seen by the physician assistant in the office on 2/1/YY for an established patient office visit ($40). Diagnosis: Bronchitis.

51 Shay Kee Hart staggers up to the window with the following charge slip. Enter these charges into the system.

CLAIM 20

Shay Kee Hart received physical therapy from Dr. Sickman for 45 minutes ($135), a whirlpool treatment ($25), and nondirect traction ($25) on 01/28/YY. The same treatments were repeated on 2/4/YY. On 2/4/YY he was also given 2.5 mg. of Methotrexate (orally) ($30). Diagnosis: Amyotrophic Lateral Sclerosis. Mr. Hart asks you to estimate his portion of the charges.

What are the total charges? _____

What is the estimated insurance payment? _____

What is the estimated patient portion? _____

Mr. Hart writes check #1835 to cover his portion of the charges (see Window Payments section). Fill in the amount of the check.

52 Return to entering Dr. Sickman's charges.

🦍 CLAIM 21

A comprehensive exam with history was performed on Cass N. O'Gen in the office ($190) on 1/29/YY. Because of a history of fibrocystic breast disease, a bilateral mammography was performed ($82). Patient complained of pelvic pain, requiring a complete pelvic ultrasound ($100). Upper respiratory infection was also diagnosed and three views of the paranasal sinuses were taken ($50). A blood specimen was collected for further testing ($15). Patient was referred to Dr. Allotta Payne, OB-GYN.

53 Dr. Goode's receptionist calls from her office and says that Al Weighs Knose is bringing his son Beane in to be looked at. She believes this family has unpaid bills from previous visits and would like to have a copy of the family's statements. Print out the statements for all family members.

Additionally, the current visit seems to require a low-complexity office visit. Let her know what the standard charge is for this service so she can collect what she can from Mr. Knose.

How much does this family still owe for previous visits? _____

How much is the standard charge for a low-complexity office visit? _____

What is the total of these two amounts? _____

Does the patient have any insurance that may cover a portion of the charges? If so, approximately how much will the insurance cover? _____

54 Dr. Goode's receptionist steps in and hands you a check from Al Weighs Knose in the amount of $75 (check #2245 [see Window Payments section]). She also hands you a charge slip for services rendered to Ron E. Knose. Enter the charges into the system.

🦍 CLAIM 22

Ron E. Knose received a low-complexity office visit ($85) and a urinalysis ($30). Diagnosis: Flu. Enter the charges into the system and apply the $75 payment to these current charges.

How much is now owed by the members of the Knose family? _____

55 The following claim information was received from Dr. Allotta Payne, OB-GYN. Enter the charges into the system.

🦍 CLAIM 23

Cass N. O'Gen received an initial consultation and comprehensive, moderate complexity visit performed at CHS Community Hospital outpatient department ($275) on 2/1/YY. Patient was referred by Dr. Yu B. Sickman. Diagnosis: Left Ovarian Mass, Pelvis Adhesions.

56 Dr. Anne S. Thesia, Anesthesiologist, provided anesthesia during the following operations. Dr. Thesia is a new provider and will need to be added into the system. Add the following information to the Provider Information screen.

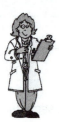

Provider:	Anne S. Thesia, M.D., Anesthesiologist
Address:	1357 Castle Blvd., Ste. 511, Colter, CO 81222
Phone:	(970) 555-3482
License #:	AST47028
EIN:	40-3445555
NPI:	1234567899
UPIN:	AST098

Provider Accepts Medicare Assignment

57 Now enter the charges provided by Dr. Thesia into the system.

CLAIM 24

Cholecystectomy with exploration of common duct ($2,550) performed on Petey Attricks on 1/15/YY. Dx: Calculus Cholecystitis. Total anesthesia time: 8:20–11:35.

CLAIM 25

A complete stripping of long, saphenous vein right leg ($1,000) performed on Sherry Attricks on 2/1/YY. Dx: Venous Insufficiency, Varicose Veins. Total anesthesia time: 9:55–11:30.

58 Print a set of day sheets or daily journal.

59 Print or write up a deposit slip for all monies received. Attach all checks and cash payments to it.

60 Reconcile petty cash. Count all money remaining in petty cash and be sure you have the same amount left at the end of the day as you started with at the beginning. If not, determine exactly where the missing amount is.

61 Print all the claims you have entered today. If you are using one-part forms, print two copies (see following exercise).

62 Prepare claims for mailing. Place one copy of the claim in the patient file. Place the second copy together with all claims for a single carrier. Print or write address labels and attach them to the claims. Place these in the folder for completed insurance claims.

63 Patient statements for the month of January need to be mailed out. Print patient statements for all patients with balances over $1.

64 Is any additional information or confirmation needed for today's transactions? If so, what?

_____

_____

_____

65 Stop and check that all assignments are correct before continuing on to the next date.

MARCH 4, CCYY

66 Today's date is March 4, CCYY. Change the date in the computer to March 4, CCYY.

67 Count petty cash. How much is in the cash envelope? _____

68 The following claim information was received from Dr. Allotta Payne, OB-GYN. Enter the charges into the system.

CLAIM 26

Cass N. O'Gen was scheduled for surgery at CHS Community Hospital on 2/12/YY. Dr. Allotta Payne, OB-GYN, performed a hysterectomy ($1,250), oophorectomy ($750), laparoscopy with lysis of adhesions ($785), dilation of vagina under anesthesia ($175), and D&C ($275). Diagnosis: Left Ovarian Mass, Pelvic Adhesions, Severe Recto-Cystocele. First seen: 1/29/YY.

69 Checks from three insurance carriers are received in the mail (Documents 22–24). Credit the appropriate amounts to the correct accounts, and then do any balance billing to either the patient or an additional insurance carrier. When billing a secondary insurance payor, be sure to attach a copy of the EOB. Data for other patients should be redacted (sensitive or classified information from a document should be removed prior to its release). A copy of the EOB need not be attached when you are balance billing the patient. The insurance carrier should have already sent them a copy of the EOB.

70 Sue Pervisor asks you for an insurance aging report. Print out the report. This will be used to contact insurance carriers who have not made payment on claims submitted over 30 days or more.

71 Checks come in from two patients (Document 25). Credit the proper accounts, and then do any balance billing to either the patient or an additional insurance carrier. When billing a secondary insurance payor, be sure to attach a copy of the EOB. Data for other patients should be redacted. A copy of the EOB need not be attached when you are balance billing the patient. The insurance carrier should have already sent them a copy of the EOB.

72 Al Weighs Knose steps up to the window with his nose in the air and a charge slip in his hand. Enter the charges into the system.

👤 CLAIM 27

Beane Andy Knose was brought into Dr. Goode's office today complaining of "something in my nose." Upon examination, a kidney bean was removed from the right nostril ($360). During examination the doctor also noted excessive earwax, which resulted in ear lavage ($80).

Al Weighs Knose writes a check (#2261) for $50 for these services (see Window Payments section). Enter the payment for $50 and print out a receipt.

73 The following claim information was received from Dr. Will Kutteroff, Surgeon. Enter the charges into the system.

📷 CLAIM 28

Carla Poole received a comprehensive consultation of moderate complexity ($275) on 2/1/YY. It was determined that she needed a bone cyst excised from the humerus ($910) and an excision of olecranon bursa ($255). These were done at CHS Community Hospital's outpatient department on 2/7/YY. Carla was referred by Dr. Sickman. Diagnosis: Tennis Elbow, Bursitis of Elbow.

74 Dr. Manny Kutz assisted with the following surgeries. Dr. Kutz is notorious for not including diagnoses and other pertinent data on his charge slips. Check the previous claims and the patient chart for any missing information. Enter the charges into the system.

👤 CLAIM 29

Cholecystectomy with exploration of common duct ($350) performed on Petey Attricks at CHS Community Hospital on 1/15/YY.

👤 CLAIM 30

Complete stripping of long, saphenous vein ($125) performed on Sherry Attricks on 2/1/YY.

👤 CLAIM 31

Hysterectomy ($150), oophorectomy ($250), a laparoscopy with lysis of adhesions ($65), and dilation of vagina under anesthesia ($35) were performed on Cass N. O'Gen on 2/12/YY. Diagnosis: Left Ovarian Mass, Pelvic Adhesions, Severe Recto-Cystocele.

75 Dr. Anne S. Thesia, Anesthesiologist, provided anesthesia during the following operation. Enter these charges into the system.

CLAIM 32
Excision of bone cyst from the humerus ($1,890) and an excision of olecranon bursa ($250) performed on Carla Poole on 2/7/YY. Diagnosis: Tennis Elbow, Bursitis of Elbow. Total anesthesia time: Start 8:50. Stop 12:35.

CLAIM 33
Vaginal hysterectomy with oophorectomy ($2,850) performed on Cass N. O'Gen on 2/12/YY. Diagnosis: Left ovarian mass, pelvic adhesions, severe recto-cystocele. Total anesthesia time: 16:10–19:25.

76 The following claim information was received from Dr. Phil Goode. Enter these charges into the system.

CLAIM 34
Dr. Goode performed a comprehensive exam of high complexity ($190) on Pat O'Gen in the office on 2/9/YY. Dr. Goode found the patient to have a cystic lesion of the left-upper eyelid and performed an outpatient excision of lesion with flap reconstruction, eyelid ($1,250) at CHS Community Hospital outpatient department on 2/12/YY. A follow-up problem-focused exam was done on 2/16/YY.

77 The following claim information was received from Dr. Yu B. Sickman. Enter these charges into the system.

CLAIM 35
Sherry Attricks requested surgery for varicose veins of the right leg. A complete stripping of long, saphenous vein ($600) was performed on 2/1/YY by Dr. Yu B. Sickman at the outpatient department of CHS Community Hospital. On 2/12/YY an injection of solution (multiple) into telangiectasia ($240) was performed by Dr. Sickman at the office. (No SSO performed.)

CLAIM 36
Scarlet Fever has not been feeling well since she went hiking with her family on 1/21/YY. She is weak with muscular aches and severe headaches and chills. On 1/27/YY, Dr. Sickman performed an office visit of high complexity ($190), CBC ($20), and WBC (manual) ($20). Dr. Sickman also gave her an injection of antibiotics ($30). Diagnosis: Rocky Mountain Spotted Fever. Patient was admitted to CHS Community Hospital on 01/28/YY.

CLAIM 37
Dr. Sickman performed an initial comprehensive H&P of high complexity on 1/28/YY ($143). Dr. Sickman also performed high-complexity hospital visits on Scarlet Fever on 1/29/YY, 1/30/YY, 1/31/YY, and 2/1/YY ($130 each). A hospital discharge was performed on 2/2/YY ($115). Diagnosis: Rocky Mountain Spotted Fever.

78 You receive an EOMB for charges with Medicare (Document 26). Enter the payments on the appropriate patient records, calculate the write-off amount and enter it into the computer. Then balance bill the appropriate party, either additional insurance or the patient if necessary.

79 Print a set of day sheets.

80 Print or write up a deposit slip for all monies received. Attach all checks and cash payments to it.

81 Reconcile petty cash. Count all money remaining in petty cash and be sure you have the same amount left at the end of the day as you started with at the beginning. If not, determine exactly where the missing amount is.

82 Print all the claims you have entered today. If you are using one-part forms, print two copies (see following exercise).

83 Prepare claims for mailing. Place one copy of the claim in the patient file. Place the second copy together with all claims for a single carrier. Print or write address labels and attach them to the claims. Be sure to separate out any claims that are for secondary insurance. They should not be billed until the EOB is received from the first carrier.

84 Print a transaction journal report. Use 3/4/YY as the date of the report. The report should include all entries, so 01/01/YY–03/04/YY should be the range of dates. This will allow the computer to pick up all entries. Check your answers before proceeding. If there are any errors, correct them.

85 Patient statements for the month of February need to be mailed out. Print patient statements for all patients with balances above $1.

86 Is any additional information or confirmation needed for today's transactions? If so, what?

_____

_____

_____

_____

Congratulations, you have now completed the simulated work portion of the course! You are now ready to prepare your resume and enter the exciting world of medical billing. **Good Luck!**

Clues For Simulated Work Program Assignments

The following clues may help you with the critical-thinking exercises contained in the simulated work program. Before looking at these clues you should attempt to answer the question on your own. Then look at the clue and determine if you should revise your answer or if you are happy with it the way it is.

Item #	Clues
15.	Are any of these diagnoses work-related?
16.	Should you tell the doctor? What options are available for payments?
34.	Consider Medicare eligibility guidelines.
36.	What would Medicare say? Are there any legal ramifications to this arrangement?
37.	Can you still bill Medicare for these charges? What are the rules?
60.	Is there a clinical person available to answer his questions? What about general available information? Other resources?
92.	Why might it make a difference what day the surgery is scheduled?
101.	How can you be sure that it arrives this time? Is there anyone you should talk to about the problem?

PATIENT INFORMATION SHEET

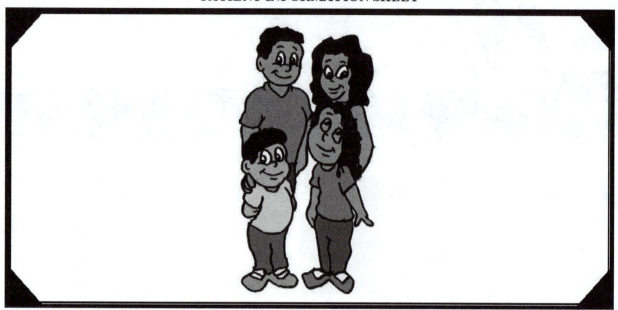

INSURED'S INFORMATION

Patient Account #: *CHS5508-001*   Assigned Provider: _____   Birth Date: *Aug. 18, CCYY-43*

Name: (Last, First, Middle) *O'Gen, Pat N.*   Gender: *Female*

Address: (Inc City, State, Zip) *621 Cayhill Ave., Colter, CO 81222*

Home Phone: *(970) 555-3311*   Marital Status: *Married*   Social Security #: *333-33-3333*

Employer Name: *White Corporation*   Work Phone: *(970) 555-1234 x591*

Employer Address: *1234 Whitaker Lane, Colter, CO 81250*   Cell Phone: *(970) 555-0002*

Employment Status: *Full-time*   Referred by: _____

Allergies/Medical Conditions: _____   Email Address: *po'gen@outofair.com*

Primary Ins Policy: *Winter Insurance Co./White Corp*   Address: *9763 Western Way, Whittier, CO 82963*

Member's ID #: *333-11 WHI*   Group Policy #: *54321*   Insured's Name: *Pat O'Gen*

Secondary Ins Policy: *N/A*   Address: _____

Member's ID #: _____   Group Policy #: _____   Insured's Name: _____

SPOUSE'S INFORMATION

Patient Account #: *CHS5508-002*   Assigned Provider: _____   Birth Date: *Nov. 12, CCYY-41*

Name: (Last, First, Middle) *O'Gen, Carson*   Gender: *Male*

Social Security #: *331-32-3334*   Employment Status: _____

Employer Name: *Self Employed*   Work Phone: _____

Employer Address: *621 Cayhill Ave., Colter, CO 81222*

Allergies/Medical Conditions: _____

Primary Ins Policy: *Winter Insurance Co./White Corp.*   Address: *9763 Western Way, Whittier, CO 82963*

Member's ID #: *333-11 WHI*   Group Policy #: *54321*   Insured's Name: *Pat O'Gen*

Secondary Ins Policy: *N/A*   Address: _____

Member's ID #: _____   Group Policy #: _____   Insured's Name: _____

CHILD #1

Patient Account #: _CHS5508-003_   Assigned Provider: _____   Birth Date: _Feb. 17, CCYY-20_

Name of Minor Child: _O'Gen, Cass N._   Social Security #: _303-17-1980_

Gender: _Female_   Marital Status: _Single_   Relationship to Insured: _Daughter_

Allergies/Medical Conditions: _____   Student Status: _Full-time student_

Primary Ins Policy: _Winter Insurance Co./White Corp._   Primary Insured: _Mother_

Secondary Ins Policy: _N/A_   Secondary Insured: _____

CHILD #2

Patient Account #: _CHS5508-004_   Assigned Provider: _____   Birth Date: _Feb. 11, CCYY-10_

Name of Minor Child: _O'Gen, Ox_   Social Security #: _198-90-2114_

Gender: _Male_   Marital Status: _Single_   Relationship to Insured: _Son_

Allergies/Medical Conditions: _____   Student Status: _Full-time student_

Primary Ins Policy: _Winter Insurance Co./White Corp._   Primary Insured: _Mother_

Secondary Ins Policy: _N/A_   Secondary Insured: _____

CHILD #3

Patient Account #: _____   Assigned Provider: _____   Birth Date: _____

Name of Minor Child: _____   Social Security #: _____

Gender: _____   Marital Status: _____   Relationship to Insured: _____

Allergies/Medical Conditions: _____   Student Status: _____

Primary Ins Policy: _____   Primary Insured: _____

Secondary Ins Policy: _____   Secondary Insured: _____

EMERGENCY CONTACT

Name: _C. R. Y. O'Gen_   Home Phone: _(970) 555- 4139_   Other Phone: _(970) 555-3406_

Address: (Inc City, State, Zip) _____ _6548 Outofair Ave. Apt# A1,3 Colter, CO 81222_

ACKNOWLEDGMENT AND AUTHORITY FOR TREATMENT AND PAYMENT

_PO_   I consent to treatment as necessary or desirable to the care of the patient(s) named above, including but not restricted to whatever drugs, medicine, performance of operations and conduct of laboratory, x-ray, or other studies that may be used by the attending doctor, his/her nurse or qualified designate:

_PO_   I also acknowledge full responsibility for the payment of such services and agree to pay for them upon demand, in full, AT THE TIME OF SERVICE. If the physician must use a collection agency/attorney or court to collect its charges, then I will pay reasonable attorney fees and costs incurred in collecting same, regardless of insurance coverage.

_PO_   I hereby authorize payment directly to Consolidated Health Services of the medical expense benefits otherwise payable to me but not to exceed my indebtedness to said physician on account of the enclosed charge.

_PO_   I hereby authorize any medical practitioner, medical or medically related facility, insurance or reinsuring company, consumer reporting agency, or employer having information with respect to any physical or mental condition and/or treatment of me or my minor children and any other nonmedical information of me and my minor children to give to the group policyholder, my employer, or its legal representative, any and all such information.

_PO_   I understand the information obtained by the use of the Authorization will be used to determine eligibility for insurance, and eligibility for benefits under any existing policy. Any information obtained will not be released by/to any organization EXCEPT to the group policyholder, my employer, reinsuring companies, the Medical Information Bureau, Inc., or other persons or organizations performing business or legal services in connection with my application, claim, or as may be otherwise lawfully required or as I may further authorize.

_PO_   I further agree that a photographic copy of this Authorization shall be valid as the original. This Authorization shall be valid for one year from the date shown below.

Signature of Insured: _Pat N. O'Gen_   Date: _Jan. 14, CCYY_

Signature of Spouse: _____   Date: _____

Document **2**

PROVIDER INFORMATION

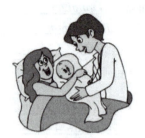

1. Provider: Allota Payne, M.D., Obstetrics and Gynecology
   Address: 1357 Castle Blvd, Ste. 500
                Colter, CO 81222
   Phone: (970) 555-5123
   License #:   AA163615
   EIN: 40-2233445
   NPI: 34562122222
   UPIN: A34621
   Provider Accepts Medicare Assignment

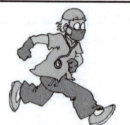

2. Provider: Phil Goode, M.D., General Practitioner
   Address: 1357 Castle Blvd, Ste. 501B
                Colter, CO 81222
   Phone: (970) 555-8425
   License #:   BB646545
   EIN: 40-2224096
   NPI: 6215033333
   UPIN: B62150
   Provider Does Not Accept Medicare Assignment

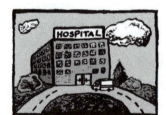

3. Provider: CHS Community Hospital
   Address: 9876 Clinton Avenue
                Colter, CO 81222
   Phone: (970) 555-9215
   License #:   HO456565
   EIN: 40-9999999
   NPI: 5321844444
   UPIN: D53218
   Provider Accepts Medicare Assignment

3a. Provider: CHS Urgent Care Trauma Center
    Address: 9800 Clinton Avenue
                Colter, CO 81222
    Phone: (970) 555-9222
    License #: TC41414
    EIN: 40-8888888
    NPI: 2468055555
    UPIN: E24680
    Provider Accepts Medicare Assignment

Provider #3 and #3a should also be entered into the address information screen becasuse doctors may provide services at this facility. Go into the Address Information screen. Use the address code CHS.

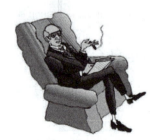

4. Provider: Reed Mi Mind, M.D., Psychiatrist
   Address: 1357 Castle Blvd, Ste. 503
                Colter, CO 81222
   Phone: (970) 555-2145
   License #:   DD484834
   EIN: 40-6666666
   NPI: 9876066666
   UPIN: F98760
   Provider Accepts Medicare Assignment

Document **3**

OFFICE VISIT PROCEDURES

DESCRIPTION	TIME	CHARGE	CPT® CODE	COST
NEW PATIENT OFFICE VISITS				
Problem-focused history/exam, straightforward	20 min	$ 65	_____	0
Expanded history/exam, straightforward	30 min	$ 85	_____	0
Detailed history/exam, low complexity	40 min	$105	_____	0
Comprehensive history/exam, moderate complexity	45 min	$115	_____	0
Comprehensive history/exam, high complexity	60 min	$135	_____	0
ESTABLISHED PATIENT OFFICE VISITS				
Minimal visit	10 min	$ 35	_____	0
Problem-focused history/exam, straightforward	15 min	$ 55	_____	0
Expanded history/exam, low complexity	20 min	$ 65	_____	0
Detailed history/exam, moderate complexity	25 min	$ 80	_____	0
Comprehensive history/exam, high complexity	30 min	$ 95	_____	0
Matrixectomy	30 min	$200	_____	45
EKG, 12 leads c/interp & report	20 min	$100	_____	15
Direction/Overseeing of emergency medical systems	15 min	$ 65	_____	10
Urinalysis	5 min	$ 30	_____	5
Specimen handling fee	5 min	$ 15	_____	0
Removal of .5 cm skin mole on neck with biopsy	45 min	$400	_____	30

ICD-9-CM CODES

Code the following diagnoses and enter the information into the Diagnosis Information screen. If necessary, add in additional descriptive information regarding the diagnosis.

	CODE	OFFICIAL CPT® DESCRIPTION
Abrasions, leg	_____	_____
Acute UTI	_____	_____
Broken Medial Ulna	_____	_____
Chest Pain	_____	_____
Chicken Pox	_____	_____
Clubfoot, congenital	_____	_____
Chronic Bronchitis	_____	_____
Concussion	_____	_____
Contusions, head	_____	_____
Cut Finger	_____	_____
Diabetes Mellitus	_____	_____
Flu	_____	_____
Gangrene	_____	_____
Hemorrhoids	_____	_____
Hyperlipidemia	_____	_____
Mole (skin), neck	_____	_____
Ovarian Mass	_____	_____
Pelvic Pain	_____	_____
Pelvis Adhesions	_____	_____
Pilonidal Cyst	_____	_____
Pregnancy	_____	_____
URI	_____	_____

Document **5**

PATIENT INFORMATION SHEET

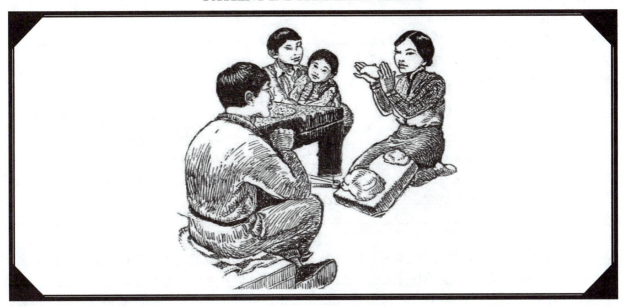

INSURED'S INFORMATION

Patient Account #: _CHS5503-001_   Assigned Provider: _Dr. Phil Goode_   Birth Date: _Apr. 4, CCYY-38_

Name: (Last, First, Middle) _Dunnitt, D. Jobb_   Gender: _Male_

Address: (Inc City, State, Zip) _160 Abernathy Ave. Apt #A, Armstrong, CO 81569_

Home Phone: _(970) 555-1122_   Marital Status: _Widowed_   Social Security #: _111-11-1111_

Employer Name: _White Corporation_   Work Phone: _(970) 555-1234_

Employer Address: _1234 Whitaker Lane, Colter, CO 81250_   Cell Phone: _(970) 555-0000_

Employment Status: _Full-time_   Referred by: _Friend-Amanda Alexander_

Allergies/Medical Conditions: _Bronchitis_   Email Address: _djobb@badcough.com_

Primary Ins Policy: _Winter Insurance Co./White Corp_   Address: _9763 Western Way, Whittier, CO 82963_

Member's ID #: _111-11 WHI_   Group Policy #: _54321_   Insured's Name: _D. Jobb Dunnitt_

Secondary Ins Policy: _N/A_   Address: _____

Member's ID #: _____ Group Policy #: _____ Insured's Name: _____

SPOUSE'S INFORMATION

Patient Account #: _____ Assigned Provider: _____ Birth Date: _____

Name: (Last, First, Middle) _N/A_   Gender: _____

Social Security #: _____ Employment Status: _____

Employer Name: _____   Work Phone: _____

Employer Address: _____

Allergies/Medical Conditions: _____

Primary Ins Policy: _____   Address: _____

Member's ID #: _____ Group Policy #: _____ Insured's Name: _____

Secondary Ins Policy: _____   Address: _____

Member's ID #: _____ Group Policy #: _____ Insured's Name: _____

CHILD #1

Patient Account #: _CHS5503-003_   Assigned Provider: _Dr. Phil Goode_   Birth Date: _Apr. 16, CCYY-14_

Name of Minor Child: _Dunnitt, Candy_   Social Security #: _104-16-1984_

Gender: _Female_   Marital Status: _Single_   Relationship to Insured: _Daughter_

Allergies/Medical Conditions: _Diabetes_   Student Status: _Full-time student_

Primary Ins Policy: _Winter Insurance Co./White Corp._   Primary Insured: _Father_

Secondary Ins Policy: _N/A_   Secondary Insured: _____

CHILD #2

Patient Account #: _CHS5503-004_   Assigned Provider: _Dr. Phil Goode_   Birth Date: _Aug. 24, CCYY-12_

Name of Minor Child: _Dunnitt, D. I._   Social Security #: _108-24-1986_

Gender: _Male_   Marital Status: _Single_   Relationship to Insured: _Son_

Allergies/Medical Conditions: _____   Student Status: _Full-time student_

Primary Ins Policy: _Winter Insurance Co./White Corp._   Primary Insured: _Father_

Secondary Ins Policy: _N/A_   Secondary Insured: _____

CHILD #3

Patient Account #: _CHS5503-005_   Assigned Provider: _Dr. Phil Goode_   Birth Date: _Oct. 16, CCYY-10_

Name of Minor Child: _Dunnitt, V. Iris_   Social Security #: _110-16-1988_

Gender: _Female_   Marital Status: _Single_   Relationship to Insured: _Daughter_

Allergies/Medical Conditions: _____   Student Status: _Full-time student_

Primary Ins Policy: _Winter Insurance Co./White Corp._   Primary Insured: _Father_

Secondary Ins Policy: _N/A_   Secondary Insured: _____

EMERGENCY CONTACT

Name: _D. Boss_   Home Phone: _(970) 555-8890_   Other Phone: _(970) 555-6031_

Address: (Inc City, State, Zip) _4310 Nowayout St., Armstrong, CO 81569_

ACKNOWLEDGMENT AND AUTHORITY FOR TREATMENT AND PAYMENT

_DD_ I consent to treatment as necessary or desirable to the care of the patient(s) named above, including but not restricted to whatever drugs, medicine, performance of operations and conduct of laboratory, x-ray, or other studies that may be used by the attending doctor, his/her nurse or qualified designate:

_DD_ I also acknowledge full responsibility for the payment of such services and agree to pay for them upon demand, in full, AT THE TIME OF SERVICE. If the physician must use a collection agency/attorney or court to collect its charges, then I will pay reasonable attorney fees and costs incurred in collecting same, regardless of insurance coverage.

_DD_ I hereby authorize payment directly to Consolidated Health Services of the medical expense benefits otherwise payable to me but not to exceed my indebtedness to said physician on account of the enclosed charge.

_DD_ I hereby authorize any medical practitioner, medical or medically related facility, insurance or reinsuring company, consumer reporting agency, or employer having information with respect to any physical or mental condition and/or treatment of me or my minor children and any other nonmedical information of me and my minor children to give to the group policyholder, my employer, or its legal representative, any and all such information.

_DD_ I understand the information obtained by the use of the Authorization will be used to determine eligibility for insurance, and eligibility for benefits under any existing policy. Any information obtained will not be released by/to any organization EXCEPT to the group policyholder, my employer, reinsuring companies, the Medical Information Bureau, Inc., or other persons or organizations performing business or legal services in connection with my application, claim, or as may be otherwise lawfully required or as I may further authorize.

_DD_ I further agree that a photographic copy of this Authorization shall be valid as the original. This Authorization shall be valid for one year from the date shown below.

Signature of Insured: _D. Job Dunnitt_   Date: _Jan. 9, CCYY_

Signature of Spouse: _____   Date: _____

Document 6

PATIENT INFORMATION SHEET

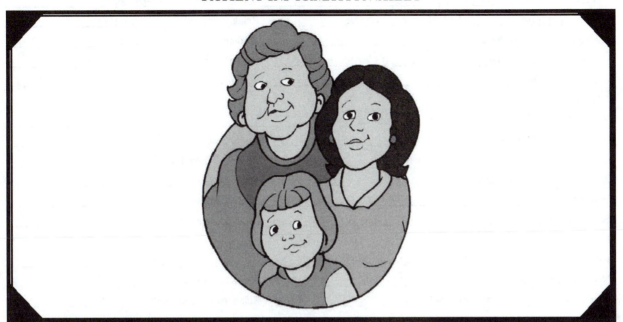

INSURED'S INFORMATION

Patient Account #: _CHS5509-001_   Assigned Provider: _____   Birth Date: _Mar. 12, CCYY-30_

Name: (Last, First, Middle) _Pendent, Codie_   Gender: _Female_

Address: (Inc City, State, Zip) _1111 E. Dunphy Drive, Colter, CO 81222_

Home Phone: _(970) 555-1965_   Marital Status: _Married_   Social Security #: _444-44-3985_

Employer Name: _Red Corporation_   Work Phone: _(970) 555-0863_

Employer Address: _1234 Nockout Road, Newton, NM 88012_   Cell Phone: _(970) 555-0003_

Employment Status: _Full-time_   Referred by: _PPO List_

Allergies/Medical Conditions: _____   Email Address: _cpendent@independent.com_

Primary Ins Policy: _Rover Insurers, Inc./Red Corporation_   Address: _5931 Rolling Road, Ronson, CO 81369_

Member's ID #: _444-44 RED_   Group Policy #: _41935_   Insured's Name: _Codie Pendent_

Secondary Ins Policy: _N/A_   Address: _____

Member's ID #: _____   Group Policy #: _____   Insured's Name: _____

SPOUSE'S INFORMATION

Patient Account #: _CHS5509-002_   Assigned Provider: _____   Birth Date: _May 15, CCYY-32_

Name: (Last, First, Middle) _Pendent, Andy_   Gender: _Male_

Social Security #: _415-19-0563_   Employment Status: _Laid Off_

Employer Name: _KDDD Radio Station_   Work Phone: _____

Employer Address: _____

Allergies/Medical Conditions: _____

Primary Ins Policy: _See Wife_   Address: _____

Member's ID #: _____   Group Policy #: _____   Insured's Name: _____

Secondary Ins Policy: _N/A_   Address: _____

Member's ID #: _____   Group Policy #: _____   Insured's Name: _____

CHILD #1

Patient Account #: _CHS5509-003_   Assigned Provider: _____   Birth Date: _Apr. 12, CCYY-7_

Name of Minor Child: _Pendent, Dee_   Social Security #: _444-01-9912_

Gender: _Female_   Marital Status: _Single_   Relationship to Insured: _Daughter_

Allergies/Medical Conditions: _____   Student Status: _Full-time student_

Primary Ins Policy: _Rover Insurers, Inc./Red Corporation_   Primary Insured: _Mother_

Secondary Ins Policy: _N/A_   Secondary Insured: _____

CHILD #2

Patient Account #: _____   Assigned Provider: _____   Birth Date: _____

Name of Minor Child: _____   Social Security #: _____

Gender: _____   Marital Status: _____   Relationship to Insured: _____

Allergies/Medical Conditions: _____   Student Status: _____

Primary Ins Policy: _____   Primary Insured: _____

Secondary Ins Policy: _____   Secondary Insured: _____

CHILD #3

Patient Account #: _____   Assigned Provider: _____   Birth Date: _____

Name of Minor Child: _____   Social Security #: _____

Gender: _____   Marital Status: _____   Relationship to Insured: _____

Allergies/Medical Conditions: _____   Student Status: _____

Primary Ins Policy: _____   Primary Insured: _____

Secondary Ins Policy: _____   Secondary Insured: _____

EMERGENCY CONTACT

Name: _N. Abor_   Home Phone: _(970) 555- 6095_   Other Phone: _(970) 555- 3569_

Address: (Inc City, State, Zip) _6518 N. Dunphy Drive Colter, CO 81222_

ACKNOWLEDGMENT AND AUTHORITY FOR TREATMENT AND PAYMENT

_CD_   I consent to treatment as necessary or desirable to the care of the patient(s) named above, including but not restricted to whatever drugs, medicine, performance of operations and conduct of laboratory, x-ray, or other studies that may be used by the attending doctor, his/her nurse or qualified designate:

_CD_   I also acknowledge full responsibility for the payment of such services and agree to pay for them upon demand, in full, AT THE TIME OF SERVICE. If the physician must use a collection agency/attorney or court to collect its charges, then I will pay reasonable attorney fees and costs incurred in collecting same, regardless of insurance coverage.

_CD_   I hereby authorize payment directly to Consolidated Health Services of the medical expense benefits otherwise payable to me but not to exceed my indebtedness to said physician on account of the enclosed charge.

_CD_   I hereby authorize any medical practitioner, medical or medically related facility, insurance or reinsuring company, consumer reporting agency, or employer having information with respect to any physical or mental condition and/or treatment of me or my minor children and any other nonmedical information of me and my minor children to give to the group policyholder, my employer, or its legal representative, any and all such information.

_CD_   I understand the information obtained by the use of the Authorization will be used to determine eligibility for insurance, and eligibility for benefits under any existing policy. Any information obtained will not be released by/to any organization EXCEPT to the group policyholder, my employer, reinsuring companies, the Medical Information Bureau, Inc., or other persons or organizations performing business or legal services in connection with my application, claim, or as may be otherwise lawfully required or as I may further authorize.

_CD_   I further agree that a photographic copy of this Authorization shall be valid as the original. This Authorization shall be valid for one year from the date shown below.

Signature of Insured: _Codie Pendent_   Date: _Jan. 1, CCYY_

Signature of Spouse: _____   Date: _____

Document 7

PROVIDER INFORMATION

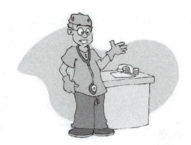

5.   Provider: Ben Dover, M.D., Gastroenterologist
     Address: 2468 Custom Blvd, Ste. 300, Colter, CO 81222
     Phone: (970) 555-6541
     License #:   FF466646
     EIN: 40-2461234
     NPI: 4900577777
     UPIN: H49005
     Provider Accepts Medicare Assignment   Rover Network Provider

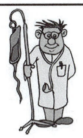

6.   Provider: Yu B. Sickman, M.D., General Practitioner
     Address: 1357 Castle Blvd, Ste. 501A, Colter, CO 812222
     Phone: (970) 555-3574
     License #:   GG369741
     EIN: 40-3759772
     NPI: 3045188888
     UPIN: I30451
     Provider Accepts Medicare Assignment

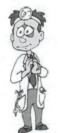

7.   Provider: Manny Kutz, M.D., Assistant Surgeon
     Address: 1357 Castle Blvd, Ste. 506, Colter, CO 81222
     Phone: (970) 555-3001
     License #:   KK987410
     EIN: 40-3159735
     NPI: 2118799999
     UPIN: L21187
     Provider Accepts Medicare Assignment

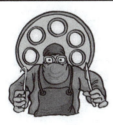

8.   Provider: Will Kutteroff, M.D., Surgeon
     Address: 1357 Castle Blvd, Ste. 507, Colter, CO 81222
     Phone: (970) 555-8652
     License #:   MM654987
     EIN: 40-9999996
     NPI: 5552500000
     UPIN: A55525
     Provider Accepts Medicare Assignment

PATIENT INFORMATION SHEET

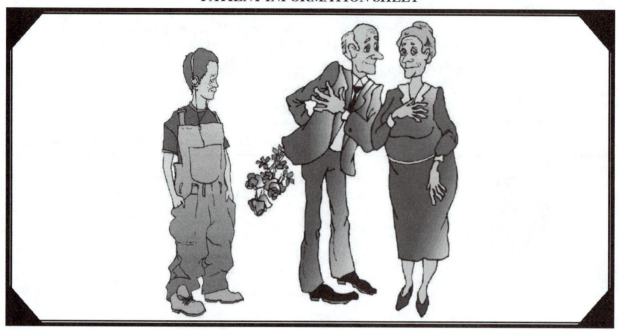

INSURED'S INFORMATION

Patient Account #: _CHS5501-001_   Assigned Provider: _____   Birth Date: _Apr. 3, CCYY-69_

Name: (Last, First, Middle) _Attricks, Jerry_   Gender: _Male_

Address: (Inc City, State, Zip) _Route 1 Box 83, Colter, CO 81235_

Home Phone: _(970) 555-5319_   Marital Status: _Married_   Social Security #: _555-23-5555_

Employer Name: _Blue Corporation_   Work Phone: _____

Employer Address: _9817 Bobcat Blvd., Bastion, CO 81319_   Cell Phone: _(970) 555-0004_

Employment Status: _Retired_   Referred by: _____

Allergies/Medical Conditions: _____   Email Address: _jattricks@pedia.com_

Primary Ins Policy: _Medicare_   Address: _1873 Montrose Ave., Minx, CO 82377_

Member's ID #: _555-23-5555A_   Group Policy #: _____   Insured's Name: _Jerry Attricks_

Secondary Ins Policy: _N/A_   Address: _____

Member's ID #: _____   Group Policy #: _____   Insured's Name: _____

SPOUSE'S INFORMATION

Patient Account #: _CHS5501-002_   Assigned Provider: _____   Birth Date: _Mar. 12, CCYY-67_

Name: (Last, First, Middle) _Attricks, Sherry_   Gender: _Female_

Social Security #: _515-51-5151_   Employment Status: _Full-time_

Employer Name: _Blue Corporation_   Work Phone: _(970) 555-9876_

Employer Address: _9817 Bobcat Blvd., Bastion, CO 81319_

Allergies/Medical Conditions: _____

Primary Ins Policy: _Ball Insurance Carriers/Blue Corp._   Address: _3895 Bubble Blvd. Ste. 283, Boxwood, CO 85931_

Member's ID #: _515-51 BLUE_   Group Policy #: _98135_   Insured's Name: _Sherry Attricks_

Secondary Ins Policy: _N/A_   Address: _____

Member's ID #: _____   Group Policy #: _____   Insured's Name: _____

CHILD #1

Patient Account #: _CHS5501-003_ _____ Assigned Provider: _____ Birth Date: _Jun. 28, CCYY-20_

Name of Minor Child: _Attricks, Petey_ _____ Social Security #: _556-19-2879_ _____

Gender: _Male_ _____ Marital Status: _Single_ _____ Relationship to Insured: _Grandchild_ _____

Allergies/Medical Conditions: _____ Student Status: _FTS Colton Community College_

Primary Ins Policy: _Ball Insurance Carrier/Blue Corp._ _____ Primary Insured: _Grandmother_ _____

Secondary Ins Policy: _N/A_ _____ Secondary Insured: _____

CHILD #2

Patient Account #: _____ Assigned Provider: _____ Birth Date: _____

Name of Minor Child: _____ Social Security #: _____

Gender: _____ Marital Status: _____ Relationship to Insured: _____

Allergies/Medical Conditions: _____ Student Status: _____

Primary Ins Policy: _____ Primary Insured: _____

Secondary Ins Policy: _____ Secondary Insured: _____

CHILD #3

Patient Account #: _____ Assigned Provider: _____ Birth Date: _____

Name of Minor Child: _____ Social Security #: _____

Gender: _____ Marital Status: _____ Relationship to Insured: _____

Allergies/Medical Conditions: _____ Student Status: _____

Primary Ins Policy: _____ Primary Insured: _____

Secondary Ins Policy: _____ Secondary Insured: _____

EMERGENCY CONTACT

Name: _Vy Agra_ _____ Home Phone: _(970) 555-5396_ Other Phone: _(970) 555-0659_

Address: (Inc City, State, Zip) _Route 2 Box 38, Colter, CO 81235_

ACKNOWLEDGMENT AND AUTHORITY FOR TREATMENT AND PAYMENT

_SA_ ___ I consent to treatment as necessary or desirable to the care of the patient(s) named above, including but not restricted to whatever drugs, medicine, performance of operations and conduct of laboratory, x-ray, or other studies that may be used by the attending doctor, his/her nurse or qualified designate:

_SA_ ___ I also acknowledge full responsibility for the payment of such services and agree to pay for them upon demand, in full, AT THE TIME OF SERVICE. If the physician must use a collection agency/attorney or court to collect its charges, then I will pay reasonable attorney fees and costs incurred in collecting same, regardless of insurance coverage.

_SA_ ___ I hereby authorize payment directly to Consolidated Health Services of the medical expense benefits otherwise payable to me but not to exceed my indebtedness to said physician on account of the enclosed charge.

_SA_ ___ I hereby authorize any medical practitioner, medical or medically related facility, insurance or reinsuring company, consumer reporting agency, or employer having information with respect to any physical or mental condition and/or treatment of me or my minor children and any other nonmedical information of me and my minor children to give to the group policyholder, my employer, or its legal representative, any and all such information.

_SA_ ___ I understand the information obtained by the use of the Authorization will be used to determine eligibility for insurance, and eligibility for benefits under any existing policy. Any information obtained will not be released by/to any organization EXCEPT to the group policyholder, my employer, reinsuring companies, the Medical Information Bureau, Inc., or other persons or organizations performing business or legal services in connection with my application, claim, or as may be otherwise lawfully required or as I may further authorize.

_SA_ ___ I further agree that a photographic copy of this Authorization shall be valid as the original. This Authorization shall be valid for one year from the date shown below.

Signature of Insured: _____ Date: _____

Signature of Spouse: _Sherry Attricks_ _____ Date: _Jan. 14, CCYY_

Appointment Calendar

DATE: *January 22, CCYY*

Time	Dr. Phil Goode	Dr. Yu B. Sickman	Dr. Allota Payne
8:00	CHS Hosp. Outpatient Dept.	Meeting	
8:15	↓	↓	
8:30	↓	↓	
8:45	↓	↓	
9:00	↓	Mal Adjusted	
9:15	↓	Sharon Needles	
9:30	↓	Anna Recksic	
9:45	↓	Di R. Rhea (10)/Mona Littlemore (5)	
10:00	↓		
10:15	↓	Wilma Leggrow-Bach	
10:30	↓	↓	
10:45	↓		
11:00	↓	Dennis Elbow (20)	
11:15	↓		
11:30	↓		
11:45	↓	Denise R. Wobbly	
12:00	↓	Lunch Mtg./Dr. Kauf	
12:15	↓	↓	
12:30	Lunch	↓	
12:45	↓	↓	
1:00	↓	↓	
1:15	↓	↓	
1:30	↓	Mary Mumps	
1:45	↓	Melissa Mumps	
2:00		Sam Manilla (25)	
2:15		↓	
2:30		Cher D. Virus (20)	
2:45			
3:00			
3:15			
3:30			
3:45			
4:00			
4:15			
4:30			
4:45			
5:00	Home	Home	
5:15	↓	↓	
5:30	↓	↓	
5:45	↓	↓	
6:00	↓	↓	

Document **10**

PATIENT INFORMATION SHEET

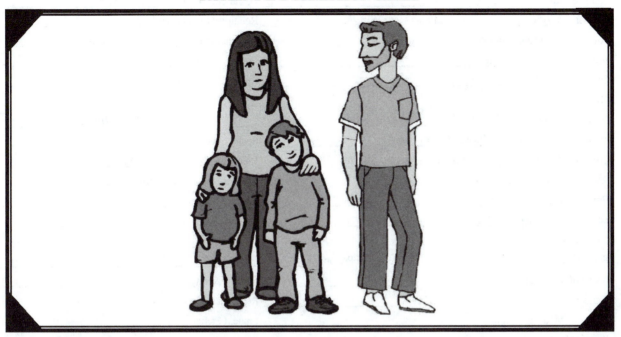

INSURED'S INFORMATION

Patient Account #: _CHS5507-001_ ___ Assigned Provider: _____ Birth Date: _Jul. 27, CCYY-34_

Name: (Last, First, Middle) _____ _Knose, Al Weighs_ _____ Gender: _Male_ ___

Address: (Inc City, State, Zip) _56789 Hamer Lane, Colter, CO 81222_ _____

Home Phone: _(970) 555-5678_ _____ Marital Status: _Married_ _____ Social Security #: _881-11-8888_ ___

Employer Name: _Self-Employed_ _____ Work Phone:_____

Employer Address: _See Above_ _____ Cell Phone: _(970) 555-0007_ ___

Employment Status: ___ _Full-time_ _____ Referred by: _____

Allergies/Medical Conditions: _____ Email Address: _awknose@clevermen.com_

Primary Ins Policy: ___ _N/A_ _____ Address:_____

Member's ID #:_____ Group Policy #: _____ Insured's Name:_____

Secondary Ins Policy: ___ _N/A_ _____ Address: _____

Member's ID #: _____ Group Policy #: _____ Insured's Name: _____

SPOUSE'S INFORMATION

Patient Account #: _CHS5507-002_ ___ Assigned Provider: _____ Birth Date: _Jan. 7, CCYY-30_

Name: (Last, First, Middle) __ _Knose, Ima_ _____ Gender: _Female_

Social Security #: __ _919-88-8598_ _____ Employment Status: ___ _Homemaker_ _____

Employer Name: __ _Self-employed_ _____ Work Phone:_____

Employer Address: _____

Allergies/Medical Conditions: _____

Primary Ins Policy: ___ _N/A_ _____ Address: _____

Member's ID #:_____ Group Policy #: _____ Insured's Name:_____

Secondary Ins Policy: ___ _N/A_ _____ Address: _____

Member's ID #: _____ Group Policy #: _____ Insured's Name: _____

CHILD #1

Patient Account #: _CHS5507-003_   Assigned Provider: _____   Birth Date: _Oct. 17, CCYY-8_

Name of Minor Child: _Knose, Ron E._   Social Security #: _810-17-8818_

Gender: _Male_   Marital Status: _Single_   Relationship to Insured: _Son_

Allergies/Medical Conditions: _Cerebral Palsy_   Student Status: _Full-time student_

Primary Ins Policy: _None_   Primary Insured: _____

Secondary Ins Policy: _N/A_   Secondary Insured: _____

CHILD #2

Patient Account #: _CHS5507-004_   Assigned Provider: _____   Birth Date: _Jun. 22, CCYY-5_

Name of Minor Child: _Knose, Beane Andy_   Social Security #: _810-22-9588_

Gender: _Male_   Marital Status: _Single_   Relationship to Insured: _Son_

Allergies/Medical Conditions: _____   Student Status: _Full-time student_

Primary Ins Policy: _None_   Primary Insured: _____

Secondary Ins Policy: _N/A_   Secondary Insured: _____

CHILD #3

Patient Account #: _____   Assigned Provider: _____   Birth Date_____

Name of Minor Child: _____   Social Security #: _____

Gender: _____   Marital Status: _____   Relationship to Insured: _____

Allergies/Medical Conditions: _____   Student Status: _____

Primary Ins Policy: _____   Primary Insured: _____

Secondary Ins Policy: _____   Secondary Insured: _____

EMERGENCY CONTACT

Name: _Noel Itall_   Home Phone: _(970) 555-2189_   Other Phone: _(970) 555-3630_

Address: (Inc City, State, Zip) _56432 Library Lane, Colter, CO 81222_

ACKNOWLEDGMENT AND AUTHORITY FOR TREATMENT AND PAYMENT

_IK_   I consent to treatment as necessary or desirable to the care of the patient(s) named above, including but not restricted to whatever drugs, medicine, performance of operations and conduct of laboratory, x-ray, or other studies that may be used by the attending doctor, his/her nurse or qualified designate:

_IK_   I also acknowledge full responsibility for the payment of such services and agree to pay for them upon demand, in full, AT THE TIME OF SERVICE. If the physician must use a collection agency/attorney or court to collect its charges, then I will pay reasonable attorney fees and costs incurred in collecting same, regardless of insurance coverage.

_IK_   I hereby authorize payment directly to Consolidated Health Services of the medical expense benefits otherwise payable to me but not to exceed my indebtedness to said physician on account of the enclosed charge.

_IK_   I hereby authorize any medical practitioner, medical or medically related facility, insurance or reinsuring company, consumer reporting agency, or employer having information with respect to any physical or mental condition and/or treatment of me or my minor children and any other nonmedical information of me and my minor children to give to the group policyholder, my employer, or its legal representative, any and all such information.

_IK_   I understand the information obtained by the use of the Authorization will be used to determine eligibility for insurance, and eligibility for benefits under any existing policy. Any information obtained will not be released by/to any organization EXCEPT to the group policyholder, my employer, reinsuring companies, the Medical Information Bureau, Inc., or other persons or organizations performing business or legal services in connection with my application, claim, or as may be otherwise lawfully required or as I may further authorize.

_IK_   I further agree that a photographic copy of this Authorization shall be valid as the original. This Authorization shall be valid for one year from the date shown below.

Signature of Insured: _____   Date: _____

Signature of Spouse: _Ima Knose_   Date: _Jan. 14, CCYY_

PATIENT INFORMATION SHEET

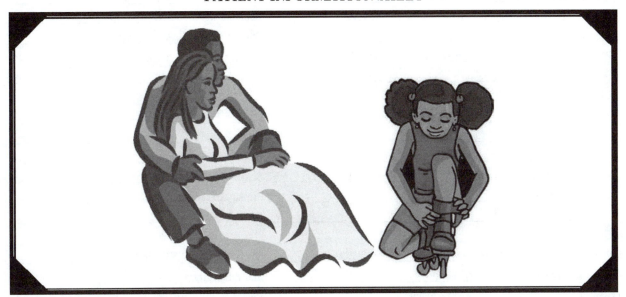

INSURED'S INFORMATION

Patient Account #: _CHS5510-001_ Assigned Provider: ___ Birth Date: _Jun. 20, CCYY-33_

Name: (Last, First, Middle) _Poole, Gene_ Gender: _Male_

Address: (Inc City, State, Zip) _4738 Jessup Road, Jasper, CO 81335_

Home Phone: _(970) 555-1335_ Marital Status: _Common Law Marr_ Social Security #: _999-99-1985_

Employer Name: _White Corporation_ Work Phone: _(970) 555-1234 x631_

Employer Address: _1234 Whitaker Lane, Colter, CO 81250_ Cell Phone: _(970) 555-0005_

Employment Status: _Full-time_ Referred by: _Co-worker_

Allergies/Medical Conditions: ___ Email Address: _gpoole@newdaddie.com_

Primary Ins Policy: _Winter Insurance Co./White Corp_ Address: _9763 Western Way, Whittier, CO 82963_

Member's ID #: _999-99 WHI_ Group Policy #: _54321_ Insured's Name: _Gene Poole_

Secondary Ins Policy: _N/A_ Address: ___

Member's ID #: ___ Group Policy #: ___ Insured's Name: ___

SPOUSE'S INFORMATION

Patient Account #: _CHS5510-002_ Assigned Provider: ___ Birth Date: _Oct. 4, CCYY-33_

Name: (Last, First, Middle) _Akenja-Nearing, Jeanette (she uses her maiden name)_ Gender: _Female_

Social Security #: _919-99-1046_ Employment Status: _Part-time_

Employer Name: _Jolly Jugglers Entertainment_ Work Phone: _(970) 555-6000_

Employer Address: _5097 Justin Way, Jasper, CO 81355_

Allergies/Medical Conditions: ___

Primary Ins Policy: _See Gene Poole_ Address: ___

Member's ID #: ___ Group Policy #: ___ Insured's Name: ___

Secondary Ins Policy: _N/A_ Address: ___

Member's ID #: ___ Group Policy #: ___ Insured's Name: ___

CHILD #1

Patient Account #: _CHS5510-003_ Assigned Provider: _____ Birth Date: _Sep. 7, CCYY-13_

Name of Minor Child: _Poole, Carla ("Car")_ Social Security #: _983-19-0907_

Gender: _Female_ Marital Status: _Single_ Relationship to Insured: _Daughter_

Allergies/Medical Conditions: _____ Student Status: _Full-time student_

Primary Ins Policy: _Winter Insurance Co./White Corp._ Primary Insured: _Mother_

Secondary Ins Policy: _N/A_ Secondary Insured: _____

CHILD #2

Patient Account #: _____ Assigned Provider: _____ Birth Date: _____

Name of Minor Child: _____ Social Security #: _____

Gender: _____ Marital Status: _____ Relationship to Insured: _____

Allergies/Medical Conditions: _____ Student Status: _____

Primary Ins Policy: _____ Primary Insured: _____

Secondary Ins Policy: _____ Secondary Insured: _____

CHILD #3

Patient Account #: _____ Assigned Provider: _____ Birth Date: _____

Name of Minor Child: _____ Social Security #: _____

Gender: _____ Marital Status: _____ Relationship to Insured: _____

Allergies/Medical Conditions: _____ Student Status: _____

Primary Ins Policy: _____ Primary Insured: _____

Secondary Ins Policy: _____ Secondary Insured: _____

EMERGENCY CONTACT

Name: _Lotta Kids_ Home Phone: _(970) 555- 0301_ Other Phone: _(970) 555- 4488_

Address: (Inc City, State, Zip) _4783 Childers Road, Jasper, CO 81335_

ACKNOWLEDGMENT AND AUTHORITY FOR TREATMENT AND PAYMENT

_GP_ I consent to treatment as necessary or desirable to the care of the patient(s) named above, including but not restricted to whatever drugs, medicine, performance of operations and conduct of laboratory, x-ray, or other studies that may be used by the attending doctor, his/her nurse or qualified designate:

_GP_ I also acknowledge full responsibility for the payment of such services and agree to pay for them upon demand, in full, AT THE TIME OF SERVICE. If the physician must use a collection agency/attorney or court to collect its charges, then I will pay reasonable attorney fees and costs incurred in collecting same, regardless of insurance coverage.

_GP_ I hereby authorize payment directly to Consolidated Health Services of the medical expense benefits otherwise payable to me but not to exceed my indebtedness to said physician on account of the enclosed charge.

_GP_ I hereby authorize any medical practitioner, medical or medically related facility, insurance or reinsuring company, consumer reporting agency, or employer having information with respect to any physical or mental condition and/or treatment of me or my minor children and any other nonmedical information of me and my minor children to give to the group policyholder, my employer, or its legal representative, any and all such information.

_GP_ I understand the information obtained by the use of the Authorization will be used to determine eligibility for insurance, and eligibility for benefits under any existing policy. Any information obtained will not be released by/to any organization EXCEPT to the group policyholder, my employer, reinsuring companies, the Medical Information Bureau, Inc., or other persons or organizations performing business or legal services in connection with my application, claim, or as may be otherwise lawfully required or as I may further authorize.

_GP_ I further agree that a photographic copy of this Authorization shall be valid as the original. This Authorization shall be valid for one year from the date shown below.

Signature of Insured: _Gene Poole_ Date: _Jan. 8, CCYY_

Signature of Spouse: _____ Date: _____

BALL INSURANCE CARRIERS   *(800) 555-5432*

3895 Bubble Blvd. Ste. 283, Boxwood, CO 85926   (970) 555-5432

| INSURANCE CONTACT: | Betty Bell | PHONE NUMBER: | (970) 555-9876 |

Policy: **BLUE Corporation, 9817 Bobcat Blvd., Bastion, CO 81319**   Insurance Group # and Suffix: **98135/BLUE**

<u>Basic/Major Medical Plan</u>   Effective 09/1/93

ELIGIBILITY EMPLOYEE: Must work a minimum of 30 hours per week. Is eligible for coverage the first of the month following three consecutive months of continuous employment.

DEPENDENTS: Are eligible for coverage from birth to age 19 or to age 23 if a full-time student or handicapped prior to age 19/23 (proof of disability must be furnished within 31 days after dependent reaches limiting age). Not eligible as a dependent if eligible as an employee. Unmarried natural children, legally adopted and foster children are included (includes legal guardianship). If both parents are covered by the plan, children may be covered by one employee only.

EFFECTIVE DATE EMPLOYEE: If written application is made prior to eligibility date, coverage becomes effective the first of the month following three months of continuous employment.

DEPENDENTS: The date acquired by the covered employee becomes the effective date if written application is made within 31 days of eligibility date. If confined in a hospital on date of eligibility, coverage will not start until the first of the month following the date the confinement ends. Newborns are automatically covered for the first 30 days following birth. Coverage will be terminated after 30 days unless written application for coverage is submitted by the employee within 31 days of birth.

TERMINATION OF COVERAGE EMPLOYEE: Coverage terminates the last day of the month following termination of employment, or when the employee ceases to qualify as an eligible employee, or following request for termination of coverage.

DEPENDENTS: Coverage terminates the date the employee's coverage terminates or the last day of the month during which the dependent no longer qualifies as an eligible dependent.

BASIC BENEFITS

PREADMISSION TESTING - Outpatient diagnostic tests performed prior to inpatient admissions; paid at 100% of UCR.

SUPPLEMENTAL ACCIDENT EXPENSE - 100% of the first $300 for services incurred within 90 days of accident.

INPATIENT HOSPITAL EXPENSE

DEDUCTIBLE: $50.
ROOM AND BOARD: 100% Up to semiprivate room charge. ICU up to $600 per day.
MISCELLANEOUS FEES: 100% Unlimited.
MAXIMUM PERIOD: Ten days per period of disability.

SURGERY

CONVERSION FACTOR: $8.50.
CALENDAR YEAR MAXIMUM: $1,600 per person.
REMARKS: Voluntary sterilizations covered.

ASSISTANT SURGERY

CONVERSION FACTOR: $8.50.
CALENDAR YEAR MAXIMUM ALLOWANCE: $320 per person. Maximum of 20% of surgeon's allowance or billed charge, whichever is less.
REMARKS: Voluntary sterilizations covered for women only.

IN-HOSPITAL PHYSICIANS

DAILY MAXIMUM: $21 for the first day; $8 per day thereafter.
MAXIMUM PERIOD: Ten days per period of disability.
REMARKS: Only one doctor can be paid per day.

ANESTHESIA

CONVERSION FACTOR: $7.50.
CALENDAR YEAR MAXIMUM: $300 per person.
REMARKS: Voluntary sterilizations covered.

OUTPATIENT PHYSICIANS VISITS

CONVERSION FACTOR: $7.50.
CALENDAR YEAR MAXIMUM: $300 per person.
REMARKS: Chiropractors, M.D.s, D.O.s and acupuncturists allowed.

X-RAY AND LABORATORY

CONVERSION FACTOR: $7.
CALENDAR YEAR MAXIMUM: $200 per person.
REMARKS: Professional component charges covered at 40% of UCR allowance for procedure. Routine procedures are not covered.

MAJOR MEDICAL EXPENSES

INDIVIDUAL CALENDAR YEAR DEDUCTIBLE:
$125; three-month carryover provision.
FAMILY MAXIMUM DEDUCTIBLE: Two family members must satisfy their individual calendar year deductible in order to satisfy the family deductible.
STANDARD COINSURANCE: 80%.
COINSURANCE LIMIT: $400 out-of-pocket per individual; $800 out-of-pocket per family (not to include deductible); aggregate.
APPLICATION OF COINSURANCE LIMIT: Coinsurance limit applies in the calendar year in which the limit is met and the following calendar year.
OUTPATIENT MENTAL/NERVOUS EXPENSE: 50% coinsurance while not a hospital inpatient.
LIFETIME MAXIMUM: $1,000,000 per person.
ROOM LIMIT: Semiprivate room rate.
HOSPITAL DEDUCTIBLE: Not covered.
HOME HEALTH CARE: 120 visits per calendar year. Prior hospital confinement required.
PREEXISTING LIMITATION: If treatment received within six months prior to effective date, $2,000 maximum payment until patient has been covered continuously under the plan for 12 months.
ANESTHESIA: Calculated using actual time.

MEDICARE

TYPE: Coordination of Benefits.
REMARKS: Assume all Medicare benefits whether or not individual actually enrolled. Subject to all other plan provisions.

EXCLUSIONS

1. Expenses resulting from self-inflicted injuries.
2. Work-related injuries or illnesses.
3. Services for which there is no charge in the absence of insurance.
4. Charges or services in excess of UCR or not medically necessary.
5. Charges for completion of claim forms and failure to keep appointments,
6. Routine or preventative or experimental services,
7. Eye refractions; contacts or glasses; orthotics (eye exercises); radial keratotomy or other procedures for surgical correction of refractive errors,
8. Custodial care,
9. Cosmetic surgery unless for repair of an injury or surgery incurred while covered or result of mastectomy,
10. Dental care of teeth, gums or alveolar process (TMJ) except: a) reduction of fractures of the jaw or facial bones; b) surgical correction of harelip, cleft palate or prognathism; c) removal of salivary duct stones; d) removal of bony cysts of jaw, torus palatinus, leukoplakia, or malignant tissues,
11. Reversal of voluntary sterilization,
12. Diagnosis or treatment of infertility including artificial insemination, in vitro fertilization, etc.,
13. Contraceptive materials or devices,
14. Nontherapeutic abortions except where the life of the mother is endangered,
15. Expenses for obesity, weight reduction, or diet control unless at least 100 lbs. overweight,
16. Vitamins, food supplements and/or protein supplements,
17. Gender-altering treatments or surgeries or related studies,
18. Orthopedic shoes or other devices for support or treatment of feet except as medically necessary following foot surgery,
19. Bio-feedback related services or treatment,
20. Experimental transplants, and
21. EDTA Chelation therapy.

COMPREHENSIVE DENTAL BENEFITS

DEDUCTIBLE: $50.
FAMILY DEDUCTIBLE LIMIT: $150; nonaggregate.
COINSURANCE: 80%.
MAXIMUM: No lifetime maximum. $1,000 per calendar year maximum.
SPACE MAINTAINER ELIGIBILITY: Employees and dependents.
FLUORIDE ELIGIBILITY: Dependents up to age 18 only.
ORTHODONTIA: No coverage.
CLAIM COST CONTROL: Predetermination of benefits and alternate course of treatment based on customarily employed methods.
PROSTHETIC REPLACEMENTS: Five-year replacement rule applies to replacements of any previously installed prosthetics.
ORDERED AND UNDELIVERED: Excludes expenses for any devices installed or delivered after 30 days following termination of insurance.
ORAL SURGERY: Covered at regular coinsurance rate, subject to calendar year maximum.
EXTENSION OF BENEFITS: 12 months.
MISSING AND UNREPLACED: Applies.

Document **13**

ROVER INSURERS, INC.
5931 ROLLING ROAD
RONSON, CO 81369
(970) 555-1369

INSURANCE CONTACT: __Ravyn Ranger__ **PHONE NUMBER:** __(970) 555-0863__

POLICY: RED Corporation, 1234 Nockout Road, Newton, NM 88012   Effective 01/01/01
INSURANCE GROUP # AND SUFFIX: 41935/RED

ELIGIBILITY EMPLOYEES must work a minimum of 30 hours per week. They are eligible for coverage the first of the month following one consecutive month of continuous employment. DEPENDENTS are eligible for coverage from birth to age 19, or to age 25 if a full-time student or handicapped prior to age 19/25. Is not eligible as a dependent if eligible as an employee. Unmarried natural children, legally adopted children, foster children, and legal guardianship children are included. If both parents are covered by the plan, children may be covered by one parent only.

EFFECTIVE DATE EMPLOYEE becomes effective, if written application is made prior to eligibility date, on the first of the month following 30 days of continuous employment. If employee is absent from work due to disability on the date of eligibility, coverage will not start until the first of the month following the date of return to active work.

DEPENDENTS become effective on the date the covered employee becomes effective, if written application is made within 31 days of eligibility date. If confined in a hospital on the date of eligibility, coverage will not start until the first of the month following the date the confinement ends. Newborns are automatically covered for the first 14 days following birth. Coverage terminates after 14 days unless written application for coverage is submitted by the employee within 31 days of birth.

TERMINATION OF COVERAGE EMPLOYEE'S coverage terminates the last day of the month following termination of employment or when the employee ceases to qualify as an eligible employee, or following request for termination of coverage. DEPENDENTS' coverage terminates the date the employee's coverage terminates, or the last day of the month during which the dependent no longer qualifies as an eligible dependent.

EXTENSION OF BENEFITS If covered under the plan when disabled, may continue coverage in accordance with COBRA. No other extension available.

COMPREHENSIVE MEDICAL BENEFITS

PREADMISSION TESTING – Outpatient diagnostic tests performed prior to inpatient admissions are paid at 100% whether through a network provider or not.

PRECERTIFICATION Voluntary, nonemergency inpatient admissions must be approved at least five days prior to admission. Emergency admissions must be precertified within 48 hrs. of admission. Benefits are reduced to 50% if not performed as required.

SECOND SURGICAL OPINION The SSO is paid at 100% of UCR. It is required for the following: bunionectomy, cataract extraction, chemonucleolysis, cholecystectomy, coronary bypass, hemorrhoidectomy, hysterectomy, inguinal herniorrhaphy, laparotomy, laminectomy, mastectomy, meniscectomy, oophorectomy, prostatectomy, salpingectomy, submucous resection, total joint replacement (hip or knee), tenotomy, varicose veins (all procedures). **IF SSO NOT PERFORMED, ALL RELATED EXPENSES PAYABLE AT 50%.**

SUPPLEMENTAL ACCIDENT EXPENSE 100% is paid on the first $500 for services incurred within 90 days of the date of accident. Subject to $20 copayment. After $500, payments are subject to calendar year deductible. Provider does not have to be a network member to receive 100% benefit. Common accident provision applies.

OUTPATIENT FACILITY CHARGES PAYABLE AT 100% - Network outpatient facility expenses for following procedures paid 100%. Does not include professional charges: arthroscopy, breast biopsy, cataract removal, bronchoscopy, deviated nasal septum, pilonidal cyst, myringotomy w/tubes, esophagoscopy, colonoscopy, herniorrhaphy (umbilical, to five years old), skin and subsequent lesions, benign and malignant (2cms+).

INDIVIDUAL CALENDAR YEAR DEDUCTIBLE $150; three-month carryover provision. All plan services subject to deductible unless otherwise indicated.

FAMILY MAXIMUM DEDUCTIBLE $300, nonaggregate. Two family members must meet individual deductible limit.

STANDARD COINSURANCE 80% for Network Providers; 60% for Nonnetwork Providers.

COINSURANCE LIMIT $1,250 out-of-pocket per individual; $2,500 out-of-pocket per family. Two individuals must meet their individual out-of-pocket limit to satisfy the family limit. Limits not to include deductible, mental/nervous expenses, or surgery expenses reduced because SSO not performed or hospital benefits reduced because precertification not performed. 100% of allowed amount paid thereafter for network providers; 80% for nonnetwork providers.

LIFETIME MAXIMUM $1,000,000 per person.

PREEXISTING LIMITATION If treatment is received within 90 days prior to effective date, no coverage on that condition for six months from the effective date (continuously covered for six consecutive months) unless treatment free for three consecutive months which ends after the effective date of coverage.

INPATIENT HOSPITAL EXPENSE   **IF NO PRECERTIFICATION, ADMISSION PAID AT 50%**

DEDUCTIBLE $200, waived for network facilities, applies to nonnetwork. Inpatient hospital expenses not subject to regular Major Medical deductible.

ROOM AND BOARD Network: 80% of semiprivate/ICU; Nonnetwork: 60% of semiprivate/ICU.

MISCELLANEOUS FEES Network Providers: 80%; Nonnetwork Providers: 60%.

EXCLUSIONS Well-baby care. Automatic coverage for first seven days if baby is ill. Otherwise, no coverage.

MENTAL/NERVOUS/PSYCHONEUROTIC

OUTPATIENT MENTAL AND NERVOUS TREATMENT

PAYABLE $60 per visit for first 5 visits; $30 per visit for next 21 visits.

COINSURANCE 80% for first five visits (maximum payable: $60 per visit), 50% per visit for next 21 visits (maximum payable: $30 per visit).

CALENDAR YEAR MAXIMUM 26 visits.

INPATIENT MENTAL AND NERVOUS TREATMENT

PHYSICIAN SERVICES 70% applies to network and nonnetwork providers.

HOSPITAL SERVICES 70% network and nonnetwork providers.

MAMMOGRAMS

COINSURANCE 80% Network Providers; 60% Nonnetwork Providers.

REQUIREMENTS Baseline mammogram for women age 35–39; for ages 40–49, one allowed every two years; for ages 50+, one allowed every year.

X-RAY AND LABORATORY PROFESSIONAL COMPONENTS Professional charges paid at 25% of UCR.

DURABLE MEDICAL EQUIPMENT

COINSURANCE 50%.

REQUIREMENTS Prescribed by M.D.; must not be primarily necessary for exercise, environmental control, convenience, comfort or hygiene. Must be an article only useful for the prescribed patient. Covered up to purchase price only.

ANESTHESIA: Use actual time.

MEDICARE

TYPE Maintenance of benefits.

REMARKS Assume all Medicare benefits whether or not individual actually enrolled. Subject to all other plan provisions.

EXCLUSIONS

1. Expenses resulting from self-inflicted injuries,
2. Work-related injuries or illnesses,
3. Services for which there is no charge in the absence of insurance,
4. Charges or services in excess of UCR or not medically necessary,
5. Preexisting conditions,
6. Charges for completion of claim forms and failure to keep appointments,
7. Routine or preventative or experimental services,
8. Eye refractions; contacts or glasses; orthotics (eye exercises); radial keratotomy or other procedures for surgical correction of refractive errors,
9. Custodial care,
10. Cosmetic surgery unless for repair of an injury or surgery incurred while covered or result of mastectomy,
11. Biofeedback related services or treatment,
12. Dental care of teeth, gums or alveolar process (TMJ) except: a) reduction of fractures of the jaw or facial bones; b) surgical correction of harelip, cleft palate or prognathism; c) removal of salivary duct stones; d) removal of bony cysts of jaw, torus palatinus, leukoplakia, or malignant tissues,
13. Reversal of voluntary sterilization,
14. Diagnosis or treatment of infertility including artificial insemination, in vitro fertilization, etc.,
15. Contraceptive materials or devices,
16. Pregnancy; pregnancy-related expenses of dependent children for the delivery including Caesarian section. Related illnesses may be covered such as pre-eclampsia, vaginal bleeding, etc.,
17. Nontherapeutic abortions except where the life of the mother is endangered.
18. Vitamins.
19. Psychological Testing.

Document **14**

WINTER INSURANCE CO, 9763 WESTERN WAY, WHITTIER, CO 82963, (970) 555-2963
POLICY: WHITE Corporation, 1234 Whitaker Lane, Colter, CO 81222 EFFECTIVE DATE: 06/01/02

INSURANCE GROUP # and SUFFIX: 54321/WHI
INSURANCE CONTACT: __Wilma Williams__   PHONE NUMBER: __(970) 555-1234__

ELIGIBILITY

EMPLOYEE: Must work a minimum of 35 hours per week. Is eligible for coverage the first of the month following 60 consecutive days of continuous employment.
DEPENDENTS: Are eligible for coverage from birth to age 19, or to age 24 if a full-time student or handicapped prior to age 19/24 (proof of disability must be furnished within 31 days after dependent reaches limiting age). Dependent is not eligible as a dependent if eligible as an employee. Unmarried natural children, legally adopted and foster children are included (also includes legal guardianship). If both parents are covered by the plan, children may be covered by one employee only.

EFFECTIVE DATE

EMPLOYEE: If written application is made prior to the eligibility date, coverage becomes effective the first of the month following 60 days of employment.
DEPENDENTS: The date acquired by the covered employee becomes the effective date if written application is made within 31 days of the eligibility date. Newborns are automatically covered for the first seven days following birth (well-baby charges excluded). Coverage will terminate after seven days unless written application for coverage is submitted by the employee within 31 days of birth.

TERMINATION OF COVERAGE

EMPLOYEE: Coverage terminates the last day of the month following termination of employment or when the employee ceases to qualify as an eligible employee, or following request for termination of coverage.
DEPENDENTS: Coverage terminates the date the employee's coverage terminates, or the last day of the month during which the dependent no longer qualifies as an eligible dependent.

EXTENSION OF BENEFITS If covered under the plan when disabled, employee may continue coverage for 12 months following the date of termination or until no longer disabled, whichever is less.

COMPREHENSIVE MEDICAL BENEFITS

SUPPLEMENTAL ACCIDENT EXPENSE 100% of first $300 for services incurred within 120 days of date of accident. Not subject to deductible.
PLAN BENEFITS
INDIVIDUAL CALENDAR YEAR DEDUCTIBLE: $100; three-month carryover provision.
FAMILY MAXIMUM DEDUCTIBLE: $200, aggregate.
STANDARD COINSURANCE: 90% except 100% of hospital room and board expenses for 365 days per lifetime.
COINSURANCE LIMIT: $750 out-of-pocket per individual; $1,500 out-of-pocket per family. Two separate members must satisfy the individual limit, not to include deductible. Applies only in the calendar year in which the limit is met.
LIFETIME MAXIMUM: $300,000 per person.
PREEXISTING LIMITATION: On 6/1/99 no restriction. After 6/1/99, if treatment received within 90 days prior to effective date, no coverage for that condition for 12 months from the effective date (continuously covered for 12 months) unless treatment free for three consecutive months ending after the effective date of coverage.

X-RAY AND LABORATORY
REMARKS: Professional component charges covered at 40% of UCR allowance for procedure. Routine procedures are not covered.

INPATIENT HOSPITAL EXPENSE
Room and board payable at 100% of semiprivate room rate. Miscellaneous expenses covered at 90%. Nonmedically necessary, well-baby care and cosmetic services excluded. Personal comfort items not covered.

MENTAL/NERVOUS/PSYCHONEUROTIC
INCLUDES SUBSTANCE ABUSE AND ALCOHOLISM.

OUTPATIENT MENTAL/NERVOUS

COINSURANCE: 50% while not hospital confined.
CALENDAR YEAR MAXIMUM: None.
INPATIENT MENTAL/NERVOUS TREATMENT
PHYSICIAN SERVICES: Covered at 90%.
HOSPITAL SERVICES: Covered at 90%.

ALLOWED PROVIDERS: Psychiatrists and clinical psychologists. Marriage and Family Child Counselor and Licensed Clinical Social Worker allowed with referral from M.D.

EXTENDED CARE FACILITY

LIFETIME MAXIMUM: 60 days.

HOSPITAL SERVICES: 80% of billed room and board charge.

REQUIREMENTS: Stay must begin within 14 days of acute hospital stay of at least three days. Extended care must be due to same disability that caused hospitalization and continued hospital care would otherwise be required.

DURABLE MEDICAL EQUIPMENT

COINSURANCE: Covered at 90%.

REQUIREMENTS: Must be prescribed by M.D. Must not be primarily necessary for exercise, environmental control, convenience, comfort, or hygiene. Must only be useful for the prescribed patient. Covered up to purchase price only.

ANESTHESIA

Computed using block time.

REMARKS

Covered expenses include charges for the initial set of contact lenses which are necessary due to cataract surgery. Handicapped children are limited to a $15,000 lifetime maximum after attainment of age 19. Coordination of Benefits according to National Association of Insurance Carriers (NAIC) guidelines. Subject to Third Party Liability and subrogation.

MEDICARE INTEGRATION

TYPE: Nonduplication of benefits applies.

REMARKS: Assume all Medicare benefits whether or not individual actually enrolled.

EXCLUSIONS

1. Expenses resulting from self-inflicted injuries, work-related injuries, or illnesses,
2. Charges or services: in excess of UCR, not medically necessary, for completion of claim forms, for failure to keep appointments; for routine, preventative or experimental services,
3. Eye refractions; contacts or glasses; orthotics (eye exercises); radial keratotomy or other procedures for surgical correction of refractive errors,
4. Custodial care and/or convalescent facility coverage,
5. Cosmetic surgery unless for repair of an injury or surgery incurred while covered or result of mastectomy,
6. Diagnosis or treatment of infertility including artificial insemination, in vitro fertilization, etc., contraceptive materials or devices, non-therapeutic abortions except where the life of the mother is endangered, reversal of voluntary sterilization,
7. Pregnancy-related expenses for dependent children.
8. Expenses for obesity, weight reduction, or diet control unless at least 100 lbs. overweight,
9. Vitamins, food supplements, and/or protein supplements,
10. Gender-altering treatments or surgeries or related studies,
11. Orthopedic shoes or other devices for support or treatment of feet except as medically necessary following foot surgery, and
12. Biofeedback-related services or treatment, EDTA chelation therapy.

COMPREHENSIVE DENTAL BENEFITS

INTEGRATED: Deductible provisions, lifetime maximum and coinsurance limit combined with comprehensive Major Medical.

CALENDAR YEAR DEDUCTIBLE: $100.

DEDUCTIBLE CARRYOVER: No carryover.

FAMILY DEDUCTIBLE LIMIT: $200, aggregate.

COINSURANCE: 90%.

COINSURANCE LIMIT: $500 (Patient responsibility, not to include disallowed amounts or the deductible.)

APPLICATION OF COINSURANCE LIMIT: Applies only in the calendar year in which the limit is met.

FAMILY COINSURANCE LIMIT: $1,000.

MAXIMUM: $300,000 lifetime.

MAXIMUM PER CALENDAR YEAR: $1,500.

ORTHODONTIA ELIGIBILITY: Dependents only.

SPACE MAINTAINER ELIGIBILITY: Dependents only.

FLUORIDE ELIGIBILITY: Employees and dependents.

ORTHODONTIC: 90% coinsurance.

ORTHODONTIC MAXIMUM: $800 lifetime; not subject to the $1,500 calendar year maximum.

CLAIM COST CONTROL OPTIONS: Predetermination of benefits required on claims over $500; alternate course of treatment based on customarily employed method. Benefits cut to 50% if no predetermination done.

PROSTHETIC REPLACEMENTS: Five-year rule applies to replacement of any previously installed prosthetics.

ORDERED AND UNDELIVERED: Excludes expenses for any devices installed or delivered after 30 days following termination date of insurance.

MISSING AND UNREPLACED EXCLUSION: Applies.

REMARKS: Orthodontic benefits are payable as incurred, rather than amortized over the period of time during which work is performed.

Document **15**

PATIENT INFORMATION SHEET

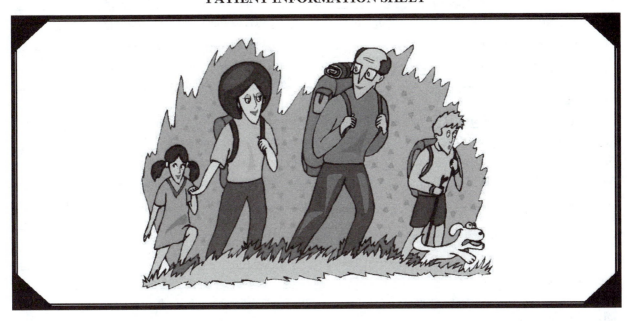

INSURED'S INFORMATION

Patient Account #: _CHS5504-001_ ___ Assigned Provider: _____ Birth Date: _Aug. 17, CCYY-53_

Name: (Last, First, Middle) _Fever, Cab N._ _____ Gender: _Male_

Address: (Inc City, State, Zip) _1432 Nightmare Way, Apt #99, Colter, CO 81352_

Home Phone: _(970) 555-1432_ _____ Marital Status: _Married_ ___ Social Security #: _014-99-1414_

Employer Name: _Red Enterprises_ _____ Work Phone: _____

Employer Address: _7677 Royal Road, Colter, CO 81293_ ___ Cell Phone: _(970) 555-0011_

Employment Status: _Full-time_ _____ Referred by: _PPO List_

Allergies/Medical Conditions: _____ Email Address: _cnfever@hightemp.com_

Primary Ins Policy: _Rover Insurers Inc/Red Enterprises_ ___ Address: _5931 Rolling Road, Ronson, CO 81369_

Member's ID #: _014-99 RED_ ___ Group Policy #: _41935_ ___ Insured's Name: _Cab N. Fever_

Secondary Ins Policy: _See Wife_ _____ Address: _____

Member's ID #: _____ Group Policy #: _____ Insured's Name: _____

SPOUSE'S INFORMATION

Patient Account #: _CHS5504-002_ ___ Assigned Provider: _____ Birth Date: _Aug. 12, CCYY-41_

Name: (Last, First, Middle) _Fever, Elle O._ _____ Gender: _Female_

Social Security #: _014-67-1764_ _____ Employment Status: _Full-time_

Employer Name: _Blue Corporation_ _____ Work Phone: _(970) 555-9876_

Employer Address: _9817 Bobcat Blvd., Bastion, CO 81319_

Allergies/Medical Conditions: _____

Primary Ins Policy: _Ball Insurance Carriers/Blue Corp_ ___ Address: _3895 Bubble Blvd. Ste. 283, Boxwood, CO 85931_

Member's ID #: _014-67 BLUE_ ___ Group Policy #: _98135_ ___ Insured's Name: _Elle O. Fever_

Secondary Ins Policy: _See Husband_ _____ Address: _____

Member's ID #: _____ Group Policy #: _____ Insured's Name: _____

CHILD #1

Patient Account #: _CHS5504-003_   Assigned Provider: _____   Birth Date: _Dec. 19, CCYY-11_

Name of Minor Child: _Fever, Scarlet_   Social Security #: _114-19-6385_

Gender: _Female_   Marital Status: _Single_   Relationship to Insured: _Daughter_

Allergies/Medical Conditions: _____   Student Status: _Full-time student_

Primary Ins Policy: _____   Primary Insured: _Father or Mother?_

Secondary Ins Policy: _____   Secondary Insured: _Father or Mother?_

CHILD #2

Patient Account #: _CHS5504-004_   Assigned Provider: _____   Birth Date: _Nov. 23, CCYY-9_

Name of Minor Child: _Fever, Ty Phoid_   Social Security #: _114-23-1740_

Gender: _Male_   Marital Status: _Single_   Relationship to Insured: _Son_

Allergies/Medical Conditions: _____   Student Status: _Full-time student_

Primary Ins Policy: _____   Primary Insured: _Father or Mother?_

Secondary Ins Policy: _____   Secondary Insured: _Father or Mother?_

CHILD #3

Patient Account #: _____   Assigned Provider: _____   Birth Date: _____

Name of Minor Child: _____   Social Security #: _____

Gender: _____   Marital Status: _____   Relationship to Insured: _____

Allergies/Medical Conditions: _____   Student Status: _____

Primary Ins Policy: _____   Primary Insured: _____

Secondary Ins Policy: _____   Secondary Insured: _____

EMERGENCY CONTACT

Name: _Hy Fever_   Home Phone: _(970) 555-3353_   Other Phone: _(970) 555-1100_

Address: (Inc City, State, Zip) _1432 Nightmare Way, Apt #95, Colter, CO 81352_

ACKNOWLEDGMENT AND AUTHORITY FOR TREATMENT AND PAYMENT

_CF_   I consent to treatment as necessary or desirable to the care of the patient(s) named above, including but not restricted to whatever drugs, medicine, performance of operations and conduct of laboratory, x-ray, or other studies that may be used by the attending doctor, his/her nurse or qualified designate:

_CF_   I also acknowledge full responsibility for the payment of such services and agree to pay for them upon demand, in full, AT THE TIME OF SERVICE. If the physician must use a collection agency/attorney or court to collect its charges, then I will pay reasonable attorney fees and costs incurred in collecting same, regardless of insurance coverage.

_CF_   I hereby authorize payment directly to Consolidated Health Services of the medical expense benefits otherwise payable to me but not to exceed my indebtedness to said physician on account of the enclosed charge.

_CF_   I hereby authorize any medical practitioner, medical or medically related facility, insurance or reinsuring company, consumer reporting agency, or employer having information with respect to any physical or mental condition and/or treatment of me or my minor children and any other nonmedical information of me and my minor children to give to the group policyholder, my employer, or its legal representative, any and all such information.

_CF_   I understand the information obtained by the use of the Authorization will be used to determine eligibility for insurance, and eligibility for benefits under any existing policy. Any information obtained will not be released by/to any organization EXCEPT to the group policyholder, my employer, reinsuring companies, the Medical Information Bureau, Inc., or other persons or organizations performing business or legal services in connection with my application, claim, or as may be otherwise lawfully required or as I may further authorize.

_CF_   I further agree that a photographic copy of this Authorization shall be valid as the original. This Authorization shall be valid for one year from the date shown below.

Signature of Insured: _Cab N. Fever_   Date: _Jan. 21, CCYY_

Signature of Spouse: _____   Date: _____

PATIENT INFORMATION SHEET

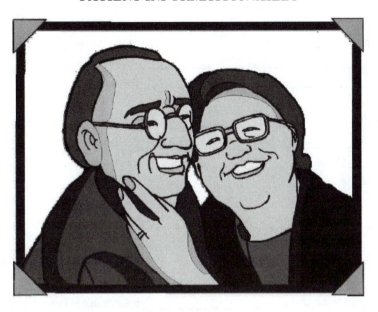

INSURED'S INFORMATION

Patient Account #: *CHS5506-001*   Assigned Provider: _____   Birth Date: *Jan. 15, CCYY-85*

Name: (Last, First, Middle) *Hart, Shay Kee*   Gender: *Male*

Address: (Inc City, State, Zip) *2093 Garden Way, Colter, CO 81223*

Home Phone: *(970) 555-9600*   Marital Status: *Married*   Social Security #: *713-77-7700*

Employer Name: *Red Enterprises*   Work Phone: *(970) 555-0863*

Employer Address: *7677 Royal Road, Colter, CO 81293*   Cell Phone: *(970) 555-0012*

Employment Status: *Retired*   Referred by: *PPO List*

Allergies/Medical Conditions: *Lou Gehrig's Disease*   Email Address: *skhart@elderlycare.com*

Primary Ins Policy: *Medicare*   Address: *1873 Montrose Ave., Minx, CO 82377*

Member's ID #: *713-77-7700A* Group Policy #: *Medigap*   Insured's Name: *Shay Kee Hart*

Secondary Ins Policy: *Rover Insurers Inc/Red Enterprises* Address: *5931 Rolling Road, Ronson, CO 81369*

Member's ID #: *713-77 RED*   Group Policy #: *41935*   Insured's Name: *Shay Kee Hart*

SPOUSE'S INFORMATION

Patient Account #: *CHS5506-002*   Assigned Provider: _____   Birth Date: *Dec. 18, CCYY-83*

Name: (Last, First, Middle) *Hart, Brooke N.*   Gender: *Female*

Social Security #: *717-71-7171*   Employment Status: *Retired Homemaker*

Employer Name: _____   Work Phone: _____

Employer Address: _____

Allergies/Medical Conditions: _____

Primary Ins Policy: *Medicare*   Address: *1873 Montrose Ave., Minx, CO 82377*

Member's ID #: *717-70-7171A* Group Policy #: _____   Insured's Name: *Brooke N. Hart*

Secondary Ins Policy: *Rover Insurers, Inc./Red Enterprises* Address: *5931 Rolling Road, Ronson, CO 81369*

Member's ID #: *713-77 RED*   Group Policy #: *41935*   Insured's Name: *Shay Kee Hart*

CHILD #1

Patient Account #: _____ Assigned Provider: _____ Birth Date: _____

Name of Minor Child: _____ Social Security #: _____

Gender: _____ Marital Status: _____ Relationship to Insured: _____

Allergies/Medical Conditions: _____ Student Status: _____

Primary Ins Policy: _____ Primary Insured: _____

Secondary Ins Policy: _____ Secondary Insured: _____

CHILD #2

Patient Account #: _____ Assigned Provider: _____ Birth Date: _____

Name of Minor Child: _____ Social Security #: _____

Gender: _____ Marital Status: _____ Relationship to Insured: _____

Allergies/Medical Conditions: _____ Student Status: _____

Primary Ins Policy: _____ Primary Insured: _____

Secondary Ins Policy: _____ Secondary Insured: _____

CHILD #3

Patient Account #: _____ Assigned Provider: _____ Birth Date: _____

Name of Minor Child: _____ Social Security #: _____

Gender: _____ Marital Status: _____ Relationship to Insured: _____

Allergies/Medical Conditions: _____ Student Status: _____

Primary Ins Policy: _____ Primary Insured: _____

Secondary Ins Policy: _____ Secondary Insured: _____

EMERGENCY CONTACT

Name: *E. K. Gee* _____ Home Phone: *(970) 555- 6452* _____ Other Phone: *(970) 555- 3008* _____

Address: (Inc City, State, Zip) *752 Forest Drive Colter, CO 81223* _____

ACKNOWLEDGMENT AND AUTHORITY FOR TREATMENT AND PAYMENT

SKH I consent to treatment as necessary or desirable to the care of the patient(s) named above, including but not restricted to whatever drugs, medicine, performance of operations and conduct of laboratory, x-ray, or other studies that may be used by the attending doctor, his/her nurse or qualified designate:

SKH I also acknowledge full responsibility for the payment of such services and agree to pay for them upon demand, in full, AT THE TIME OF SERVICE. If the physician must use a collection agency/attorney or court to collect its charges, then I will pay reasonable attorney fees and costs incurred in collecting same, regardless of insurance coverage.

SKH I hereby authorize payment directly to Consolidated Health Services of the medical expense benefits otherwise payable to me but not to exceed my indebtedness to said physician on account of the enclosed charge.

SKH I hereby authorize any medical practitioner, medical or medically related facility, insurance or reinsuring company, consumer reporting agency, or employer having information with respect to any physical or mental condition and/or treatment of me or my minor children and any other nonmedical information of me and my minor children to give to the group policyholder, my employer, or its legal representative, any and all such information.

SKH I understand the information obtained by the use of the Authorization will be used to determine eligibility for insurance, and eligibility for benefits under any existing policy. Any information obtained will not be released by/to any organization EXCEPT to the group policyholder, my employer, reinsuring companies, the Medical Information Bureau, Inc., or other persons or organizations performing business or legal services in connection with my application, claim, or as may be otherwise lawfully required or as I may further authorize.

SKH I further agree that a photographic copy of this Authorization shall be valid as the original. This Authorization shall be valid for one year from the date shown below.

Signature of Insured: *Shay Kee Hart* _____ Date: *Jan. 21, CCYY* _____

Signature of Spouse: _____ Date: _____

TYPE	PROCEDURE CODE	DESCRIPTION
A	HRDSHP	Write-off due to patient's financial hardship.
A	DEC	Amount written off due to death of patient.
A	CHG ERR	Amount changed due to an error in the original charge. This can be a negative or a positive adjustment (i.e., a lessor or higher amount added to the original charge).
A	CODE ERR	Amount changed or deleted due to an error in the procedure code entry. This adjustment would be best served by adjusting out the old charge and entering the new procedure code.
A	PT REQ	Amount adjusted due to patient demand. (This code may be used to adjust a cost if the patient is dissatisfied with service and/or insists the charge is excessive for the services rendered.)
A	CTSY FAM	Amount adjusted as a patient courtesy due to patient's familial relationship to another Consolidated Health Services provider.
A	DISC PT	Patient has discontinued treatment with this provider and there is no hope of recovering payment.
A	PT UNK	Patient address, phone, and other information are unknown (i.e., patient has moved and left no forwarding address). Efforts to trace patient have been unsuccessful.
B	INS DWNCD	Insurance downcoded charges. The insurance carrier ruled that the procedures rendered did not justify the higher code level.
B	MCR APP	Amount adjusted to conform to Medicare's approved amount.

NOTE: All providers should break down adjustments to prevent a loss of time. In an audit situation, the auditors will need to know the reason behind each of the adjustments.

WINTER INSURANCE
9763 WESTERN WAY
WHITTIER, CO 82963

PATIENT NAME	DATE OF SERVICE	PROCEDURE	BILLED AMOUNT	ALLOWED AMOUNT	% OF AMOUNT	PAYMENT AMOUNT	DENIED AMOUNT	REASON CODE
ID#: 999-99 WHI			$ 55.00	$ 50.00			$ 5.00	
O'GEN, OX	01/14/YY	OFFICE VISIT	$ 55.00	$ 50.00	90%	$ 0.00***	$ 5.00	45
ID#: 333-11 WHI								
TOTAL			$ 55.00	$ 50.00		$ 0.00	$ 5.00	
ID#: 111-11 WHI								
GRAND TOTAL			$55.00	$50.00		$0.00	$5.00	

REASON CODES:

*** APPLIED TOWARD DEDUCTIBLE

DETACH CHECK BEFORE CASHING

WINTER INSURANCE
9763 WESTERN WAY
WHITTIER, CO 82963

BANK OF COLORS
Whittier Branch
2300 Whyme Way
Whittier, CO 82963

(970) 555-5555

1111
33-77
1293

January 24, 20 YY

PAY   Zero and no/100 _____ DOLLARS $ 0.00

TO
THE
ORDER
OF

Consolidated Health Services
1357 Castle Blvd, Suite 515
Colter, CO 81222-2222

William Windsor

0123   4567   0000011123

||.001111||.:111000123:

AL WEIGHS KNOSE
56789 HAMMER LANE
COLTER, CO 81222

2230
11-00
1110

January 30   20 *YY*

Pay to the
order of   *Consolidated Health Services* | $ 50.00

Fifty and no/100-- Dollars

THE BEST BANK
9012 BAKER BLVD.
COLTER, CO 81234

For *Ron's & Ima's Dr. Visits 1/14*   *Al Weighs Knose*

:11100011: 230 0000 123456

**Jeanette Akenja-Nearing
& Gene Poole**
4738 JESSUP ROAD
JASPER, CO 81335

920
33-13
1110

January 31   20 *YY*

Pay to the
order of   *Consolidated Health Services* | $ 150.00

One Hundred Fifty Dollars and 00/100------------------------ Dollars

THIRD BEST BANK
3033 THIRD STREET
COLTER, CO 81333

For *Carla $5 and Gene $145*   *Gene Poole*

:11100011: 230 0000 123456

PAT N. O'GEN
621 CAYHILL AVE.
COLTER, CO 81222

2933
22-31
1110

January 26   20 *YY*

Pay to the
order of   *Consolidated Health Services* | $ 30.00

Thirty and no/100-- Dollars

SECOND BEST BANK
2223 SAHARA STREET
COLTER, CO 81221

For *Ox's Dr. Visit*   *Pat N. O'Gen*

:11100011: 230 0000 123456

ROVER INSURERS INC.
5931 ROLLING ROAD
RONSON, CO 81369

PATIENT NAME	DATE OF SERVICE	PROCEDURE	BILLED AMOUNT	ALLOWED AMOUNT	% OF AMOUNT	PAYMENT AMOUNT	DENIED AMOUNT	REASON CODE
PENDENT, DEE ID#: 444-44 RED	01/14/YY	OFFICE VISIT	$ 35.00	$ 35.00	80%	$ 8.00***	$ 0.00	36
GRAND TOTAL			$ 35.00	$ 35.00		$ 8.00	$ 0.00	

REASON CODES:

36   BILLED AMOUNT EXCEEDS AMOUNT ALLOWED BY THE PLAN.

*** $25 LEFT ON DEDUCTIBLE AFTER CARRYOVER DEDUCTIBLE CALCULATED

*   APPLIED TOWARD DEDUCTIBLE

DETACH CHECK BEFORE CASHING

ROVER INSURERS, INC.
5931 ROLLING ROAD
RONSON, CO 81369

BANK OF COLORS (970) 555-5555
Ronson Branch
2300 Rocky Road
Ronson, CO 81369

04-9999

08-12
1100

January 31,   20 YY

PAY   Eight and no/100   DOLLARS $ 8.00

TO
THE
ORDER
OF

Consolidated Health Services
1357 Castle Blvd, Suite 515
Colter, CO 81222-2222

Randy Rover
‖0000011123‖

‖001111‖ :111000123: 0123 4567‖

BALL INSURANCE CARRIERS
3895 BUBBLE BLVD.
BOXWOOD, CO 85926

PATIENT NAME	DATE OF SERVICE	PROCEDURE	BILLED AMOUNT	ALLOWED AMOUNT	BASIC AMOUNT	PAYMENT AMOUNT	DENIED AMOUNT	REASON CODE
ATTRICKS, PETEY	01/14/YY	OFFICE VISIT	$190.00	$148.00	8.50	$11.60***	$42.00	19
ID#: 515-51 BLUE	01/14/YY	BLOOD SAMPLE	$15.00	$7.50	.20	$5.84	$7.50	19
	TOTAL		$205.00	$155.50	8.70	$17.44	$49.50	
ATTRICKS, PETEY	01/14/YY	COMP CONSULT	$275.00	$225.00	12.75	$169.80	$50.00	19
ID#: 515-51 BLUE	TOTAL		$275.00	$225.00	12.75	$169.80	$50.00	
GRAND TOTAL			$480.00	$380.50	$21.45	$187.24	$99.50	

REASON CODES:

19   BILLED AMOUNT EXCEEDS AMOUNT ALLOWED BY THE PLAN.
*   ACCIDENT BENEFIT AMOUNT
*** APPLIED TOWARD DEDUCTIBLE

DETACH CHECK BEFORE CASHING

BANK OF COLORS (970) 555-5555   12341
Boxwood Branch   01-11
2300 Barker Blvd.   1000
Boxwood, CO 85926

                                        January 31,   20 YY

                                        DOLLARS $ 208.69

Bob Brader

0123   4567‖   ‖000011123‖

BALL INSURANCE CARRIERS
3895 BUBBLE BLVD.
BOXWOOD, CO 85926

PAY   Two Hundred Eight and 69/100

TO
THE   Consolidated Health Services
ORDER   1357 Castle Blvd, Suite 515
OF   Colter, CO 81222-2222

‖001111‖ :11000123:

ROVER INSURERS, INC.
5931 ROLLING ROAD
RONSON, CO 81369

PATIENT NAME	DATE OF SERVICE	PROCEDURE	BILLED AMOUNT	ALLOWED AMOUNT	% OF AMOUNT	PAYMENT AMOUNT	DENIED AMOUNT	REASON CODE
PENDENT, CODIE	01/17/YY	IND PSYCH	$160.00	$112.50	80%	$0.00*	$ 47.50	36
ID#: 444-44 RED	01/17/YY	PSYCH TESTING	$575.00	$ 0.00		$0.00	$575.00	91
	TOTAL		$735.00	$112.50		$0.00	$622.50	
GRAND TOTAL			$735.00	$112.00		$0.00	$622.50	

REASON CODES:
36 BILLED AMOUNT EXCEEDS AMOUNT ALLOWED BY THE PLAN.
91 PSYCHOLOGICAL TESTING IS NOT COVERED BY YOUR PLAN.
*   APPLIED TOWARD DEDUCTIBLE

DETACH CHECK BEFORE CASHING

No check issued.
Ø Balance due.

BALL INSURANCE CARRIERS
3895 BUBBLE BLVD.
BOXWOOD, CO 85926

PATIENT NAME	DATE OF SERVICE	PROCEDURE	BILLED AMOUNT	ALLOWED AMOUNT	BASIC AMOUNT	80% AMOUNT	DENIED AMOUNT	REASON CODE
FEVER, TY PHOID	01/21/YY	OFFICE VISIT	$150.00	$117.50	6.75	$0.00*	$32.50	19
ID# 014-67 BLUE	TOTAL		$150.00	$117.50	6.75	$0.00	$32.50	
GRAND TOTAL			$150.00	$117.50	$6.75	$0.00	$32.50	

REASON CODES:

19   BILLED AMOUNT EXCEEDS AMOUNT ALLOWED BY THE PLAN.
*   APPLIED TOWARD DEDUCTIBLE

DETACH CHECK BEFORE CASHING

BANK OF COLORS (970) 555-5555   **2345**
Boxwood Branch
2300 Barker Blvd.   01-11
Boxwood, CO 85926   ————
                                                                          1000

                                                   February 21,   20 YY _____

                                          DOLLARS $ 6.75

                                                   Bob Brader

0123   4567‖   ‖0000011123‖

BALL INSURANCE CARRIERS
3895 BUBBLE BLVD.
BOXWOOD, CO 85926

PAY   Six and 75/100

TO
THE   Consolidated Health Services
ORDER 1357 Castle Blvd, Suite 515
OF   Colter, CO 81222-2222

‖001111‖:111000123:

WINTER INSURANCE
9763 WESTERN WAY
WHITTIER, CO 82963

PATIENT NAME	DATE OF SERVICE	PROCEDURE	BILLED AMOUNT	ALLOWED AMOUNT	% OF AMOUNT	PAYMENT AMOUNT	DENIED AMOUNT	REASON CODE
POOLE, CARLA	01/14/YY	OFFICE VISIT	$ 85.00	$ 55.00	100%*	$ 55.00	$ 30.00	45
ID# 999-99 WHI	01/14/YY	X-RAY FINGER	$ 40.00	$ 31.00	100%*	$ 31.00	$ 9.00	45
	01/14/YY	STERILE TRAY	$ 50.00	$ 50.00	100%*	$ 50.00	$ 0.00	45
	TOTAL		$175.00	$136.00		$136.00	$ 39.00	

| GRAND TOTAL | | | $175.00 | $136.00 | | $136.00 | $ 39.00 | |

REASON CODES:

45   BILLED AMOUNT EXCEEDS AMOUNT ALLOWED BY THE PLAN.

*   ACCIDENT BENEFIT AMOUNT

DETACH CHECK BEFORE CASHING

WINTER INSURANCE
9763 WESTERN WAY
WHITTIER, CO 82963

BANK OF COLORS   (970) 555-5555   04-9999
Whittier Branch $\frac{33-77}{1293}$
2300 Whyme Way
Whittier, CO 82963

     February 26,   20 YY

PAY   One Hundred Thirty Six and 00/100**********************************   DOLLARS $ 136.00

TO
THE   Consolidated Health Services
ORDER   1357 Castle Blvd, Suite 515
OF   Colter, CO 81222-2222

                               Tom Trustee

||001111|| ⁙111000123:   0123   4567|| || 0000011123||

ANDY PENDENT   2148
1111 E Dunphy Ave   11-00
Colter, CO 81222   1110

                                                    February 23   20 *YY*

Pay to the
order of *Consolidated Health Services* | *$ 171.00*

One Hundred Seventy One and 00/100--- Dollars

THE BEST BANK
9012 BAKER BLVD.
COLTER, CO 81234

For _____   *Andy Pendent*

|:11100011|: 230 0000 123456 || ▪

SHERRY ATTRICKS   1979
RT 1 BOX 83   22-31
COLTER, CO 81235   1110

                                                    February 21   20 *YY*

Pay to the
order of *Consolidated Health Services* | *$ 100.00*

One Hundred and no/100-- Dollars

SECOND BEST BANK
2223 SAHARA STREET
COLTER, CO 81221

For *Petey*   *Sherry Attricks*

|:11100011|: 230 0000 123456 || ▪

Document **26**

MEDICARE REMITTANCE NOTICE

DATE: FEBRUARY 27, 20YY
CHECK SEQUENCE NO.: 2AF-01241351-2
PAGE 1 OF 1

BENEFICIARY NAME HIC NO EX NO	SVC FR MO-DY	TO DY-YR	PLACE TYPE	PROCEDURE DESCRIPTION	AMOUNT BILLED	AMOUNT APPROVED	SEE NOTE	DEDUCTIBLE	COINSUR.	PAYMENT	INTEREST
SHAY KEE HART	01-21	21-YY	1	OV	190.00	176.55	56				
	01-21	21-YY	1	URINALYSIS	30.00	9.91	56				
	713-77-7700A			TOTALS	220.00	186.46	442	100.00	17.29	69.17	0.00
SHAY KEE HART	01-28	28-YY	1	PHYS THER	135.00	86.82	56				
	01-28	28-YY	1	WHIRLPOOL	25.00	19.91	56				
	01-28	28-YY	1	TRACTION N/D	25.00	18.63	56				
	02-04	04-YY	1	PHYS THER	135.00	86.82	56				
	02-04	04-YY	1	WHIRLPOOL	25.00	19.91	56				
	02-04	04-YY	1	TRACTION N/D	25.00	18.63	56				
	02-04	04-YY	1	METHOTREXATE	30.00	19.95	56				
	713-77-7700A			TOTALS	400.00	270.67	442	0.00	54.13	216.54	0.00
TOTAL					620.00	457.13		100.00	71.42	285.71	0.00

56 - Medicare limits payment to this amount.
442 - Total for these charges.

DETACH CHECK BEFORE CASHING

MEDICARE	**BANK OF COLORS** (970) 555-5555	04-9999
1873 MONTROSE AVE	2300 Matchbox Way	99-123
MINX, CO 82377	Minx, CO 82377	87654

February 27, 20 YY

PAY Two Hundred Eighty Five and 71/100** DOLLARS $ 285.71

TO
THE
ORDER
OF

Consolidated Health Services
1357 Castle Blvd, Suite 515
Colter, CO 81222-2222

Mike Medicarier

⑈ .001111⑈ . #:111000123#: 0123 4567⑈ . ⑈ .0000011123⑈ .

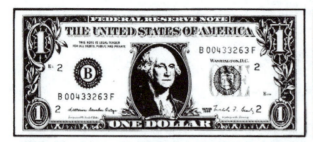
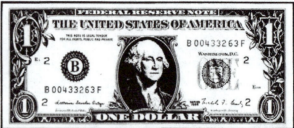

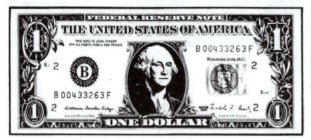
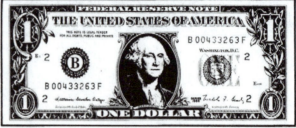

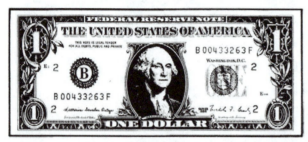
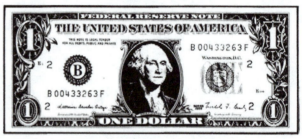

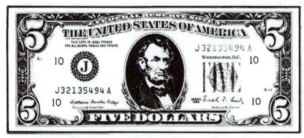
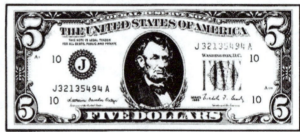

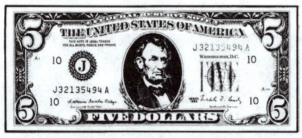
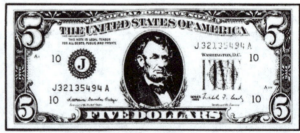

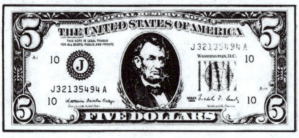
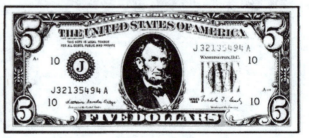

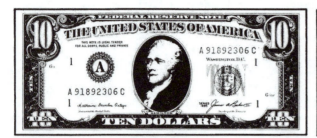

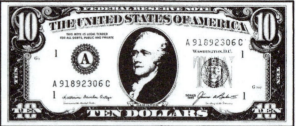

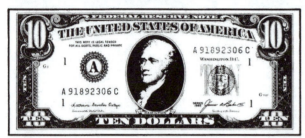

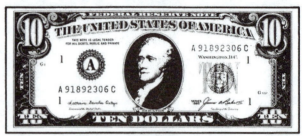

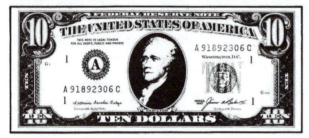

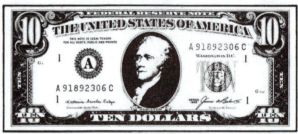

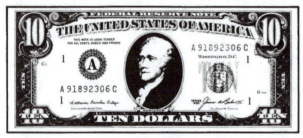

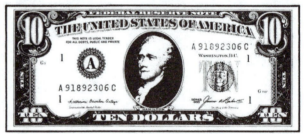

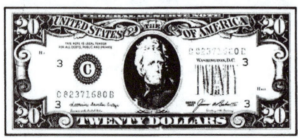

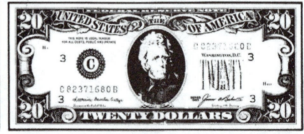

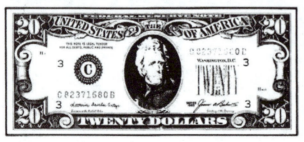

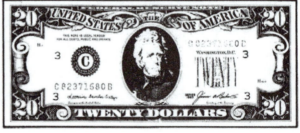

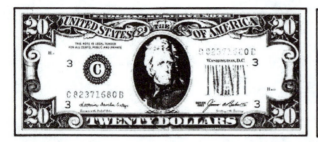
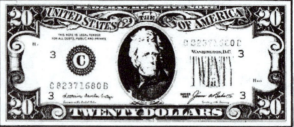
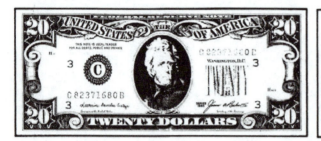
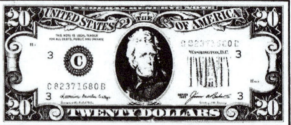
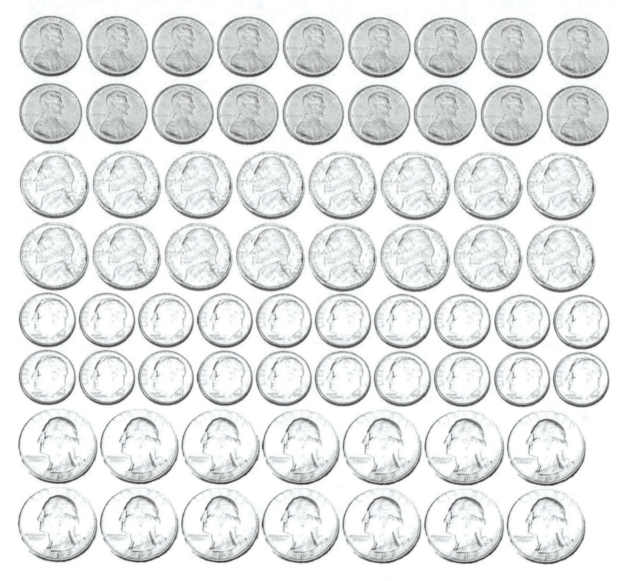

WINDOW PAYMENTS: The following payments were received at the billing office window or given with the claim information.

CLAIM 1 – Ox O'Gen

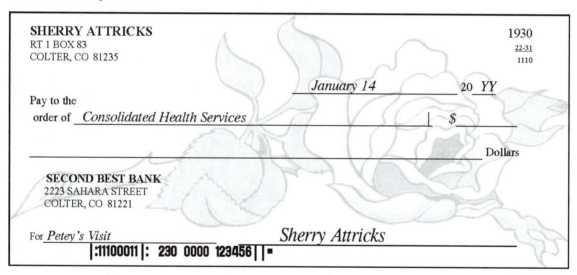

PAT N. O'GEN   2929
621 CAYHILL AVE.   22-31
COLTER, CO 81222   1110

                                          January 14   20 YY

Pay to the
order of   Consolidated Health Services $ 25.00

Twenty Five and no/100--- Dollars

SECOND BEST BANK
2223 SAHARA STREET
COLTER, CO 81221

For Ox's Dr. Visit   Pat N. O'Gen
:11100011|: 230 0000 123456|| ▪

CLAIM 3 – Petey Attricks

SHERRY ATTRICKS   1930
RT 1 BOX 83   22-31
COLTER, CO 81235   1110

                                          January 14   20 YY

Pay to the
order of   Consolidated Health Services | $

_____ Dollars

SECOND BEST BANK
2223 SAHARA STREET
COLTER, CO 81221

For Petey's Visit   Sherry Attricks
:11100011|: 230 0000 123456|| ▪

CLAIM 5 – Ima Knose   ### CLAIM 6 – Ron E. Knose

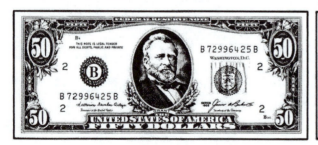   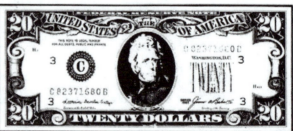

CLAIM 7 – V. Iris

D. JOBB DUNNITT   1805
160 ABERNATHY AVE #A   22-31
ARMSTRONG, CO 81569   1110

                                     January 21   20 YY

Pay to the
order of *Consolidated Health Services* $

_____ Dollars

SECOND BEST BANK
2223 SAHARA STREET
COLTER, CO 81222

For *V. Iris's 1/21/YY Dr. Visit*   *D. Jobb Dunnitt*
|:1110011|: 230 0000 123456||▪

CLAIM 10 – Shay Kee Hart

SHAY KEE & BROOKE N. HART   1796
2093 GARDEN WAY   33-13
COLTER, CO 81223   1110

                                     January 21   20 YY

Pay to the
order of *Consolidated Health Services* $

_____ Dollars

THE BEST BANK
9012 BAKER BLVD.
COLTER, CO 81234

For *Medicare Ded & Est Pmt*   *Shay Kee Hart*
|:1110011|: 230 0000 123456||▪

CLAIM 13 – Sherry Attricks

SHERRY ATTRICKS   1932
RT 1 BOX 83   22-31
COLTER, CO 81235   1110

                                     February 4   20 YY

Pay to the
order of *Consolidated Health Services* $ 45.00

Forty Five and no/100--- Dollars

SECOND BEST BANK
2223 SAHARA STREET
COLTER, CO 81221

For *Sherry's, 2/4/YY Visit*   *Sherry Attricks*
|:1110011|: 230 0000 123456||▪

CLAIM 16 – Andy Pendent

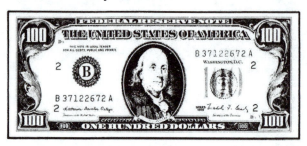

CLAIM 17 – D. Jobb Dunnitt

D. JOBB DUNNITT   1809
160 ABERNATHY AVE #A   22-31
ARMSTRONG, CO 81569   1110

                                                              January 23   20 *YY*

Pay to the
order of *Consolidated Health Services* $ *60.00*

Sixty and 00/100-- Dollars

 SECOND BEST BANK
 2223 SAHARA STREET
 COLTER, CO 81222

For *1/23/YY Hospital Visit*   *D. Jobb Dunnitt*

⑈11100011⑈ 230 0000 123456 ‖ ■

CLAIM 20 – Shay Kee Hart

SHAY KEE & BROOKE N. HART   1835
2093 GARDEN WAY   33-13
COLTER, CO 81223   1110

                                                      February 2   20 *YY*

Pay to the
order of *Consolidated Health Services* $_____

_____ Dollars

 THE BEST BANK
 9012 BAKER BLVD.
 COLTER, CO 81234

For *Est payment Dr. Visit 2/4/YY*   *Shay Kee Hart*

⑈11100011⑈ 230 0000 123456 ‖ ■

CLAIM 22 – Ron E. Knose

AL WEIGHS KNOSE   2245
56789 HAMMER LANE   11-00
COLTER, CO 81222   1110

February 4   20 YY

Pay to the
order of   Consolidated Health Services $ 75.00

Seventy Five and no/100--- Dollars

THE BEST BANK
9012 BAKER BLVD.
COLTER, CO 81234

For Ron's 2/4/YY Visit   Al Weighs Knose

|:11100011|: 230 0000 123456||■

CLAIM 27 – Beane Andy Knose

AL WEIGHS KNOSE   2261
56789 HAMMER LANE   11-00
COLTER, CO 81222   1110

March 2   20 YY

Pay to the
order of   Consolidated Health Services $ 50.00

Fifty and 00/100--- Dollars

THE BEST BANK
9012 BAKER BLVD.
COLTER, CO 81234

For   Al Weighs Knose

|:11100011|: 230 0000 123456||■

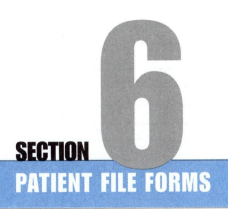

SECTION 6
PATIENT FILE FORMS

RECEIPT

DEPOSIT TICKET

PETTY CASH COUNT

PETTY CASH RECEIPT

STATIONERY

REQUEST FOR ADDITIONAL INFORMATION

INSURANCE COVERAGE FORM

RECEIPT

Date _____ CC _____ No.

ANY BILLING SERVICE
123 Any Way
Anytown, USA 12345
(123) 456-7890

Received From _____

Address _____

_____ Dollars $ _____

For _____

ACCOUNT			HOW PAID			
AMT OF ACCOUNT			CASH			
AMT PAID			CHECK			
BALANCE DUE			MONEY ORDER		By _____

DEPOSIT TICKET

ADDRESS_____

_____

DATE _____ DOLLARS   CENTS

Any Bank
Any City Branch
P.O. Box 0000
Any City, USA 90000

⑈: 123456789: 09876:: 54321

	DOLLARS	CENTS
CURRENCY		
COIN		
CHECKS 1		
2		
3		
4		
5		
6		
7		
8		
9		
10		
11		
12		
13		
14		
15		
16		
17		
18		
19		
20		
21		
22		
23		
24		
25		
26		
27		
28		
29		
30		
31		
32		
33		
34		
35		
TOTAL		

Total Deposit

DEPOSITS MAY NOT BE AVAILABLE FOR IMMEDIATE WITHDRAWAL

PETTY CASH COUNT

DATE _____

TIME _____

	QUANTITY	AMOUNT
CURRENCY		
$100	_____	_____
$50	_____	_____
$20	_____	_____
$10	_____	_____
$5	_____	_____
$1	_____	_____
TOTAL		_____
COINS		
$1	_____	_____
Half $	_____	_____
Quarters	_____	_____
Dimes	_____	_____
Nickels	_____	_____
Pennies	_____	_____
TOTAL		_____
RECEIPTS TOTAL	+	_____
GRAND TOTAL		_____

PETTY CASH RECEIPT

RECEIVED OF PETTY CASH

NUMBER _____   DATE _____

AMOUNT _____

FOR _____

_____

_____

CHARGE TO ACCOUNT _____

APPROVED BY _____   RECEIVED BY _____

Following are the file forms you will need if you are completing some or all of the Simulated Work Program in a manual format. One copy of each of the forms has been provided here. Although these forms are copyrighted by ICDC Publishing, Inc., purchase of this text allows you the right to copy these forms as needed to complete the Simulated Work Program assignments.

CONSOLIDATED HEALTH SERVICES

Medical Billing Office
1357 Castle Blvd., Suite 515
Colter, CO 81222
(970) 555-4567

Serving all your medical needs for 17 years

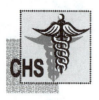

CONSOLIDATED HEALTH SERVICES

Medical Billing Office
1357 Castle Blvd., Suite 515
Colter, CO 81222
(970) 555-4567

Date: _____

Re: Policy Holder: _____

Patient Account #: _____

Employee: _____

Dependent: _____

Dear _____ :

We need additional information from you.

We are writing to _____

_____

_____

_____

_____

_____

Please respond on the reverse of this letter or attach additional information or documentation. Thank you.

Sincerely yours,

Serving all your medical needs for 17 years!

CONSOLIDATED HEALTH SERVICES
Medical Billing Office
1357 Castle Blvd., Suite 515
Colter, CO 81222
(970) 555-4567

Insurance Coverage Form

INSURED: _____ BIRTH DATE: _____

SSN: _____ EFFECTIVE DATE: _____

INSURANCE POLICY: _____

ADDRESS: _____

ID/MEMBER #: _____ GROUP #: _____

DEPENDENT AGE LIMIT: _____

_____

INDIV. DEDUCTIBLE AMOUNT: _____ 3 MO CARRYOVER:_____

FAMILY DEDUCTIBLE: _____AGGREGATE/NONAGGREGATE

STANDARD COINSURANCE:_____ LIFETIME MAXIMUM: _____

COINSURANCE LIMIT: _____

_____

BENEFITS PAID AT OTHER THAN THE STANDARD COINSURANCE % [Including benefit, coinsurance amount and special circumstances (i.e., SSO allowed at 100%, required for hysterectomy, coronary bypass, etc.)]:

_____

_____

PREAUTHORIZATION REQUIRED FOR: _____

_____

ACCIDENT BENEFIT AMOUNT: _____ TREATMENT TO BE RECEIVED WITHIN _____ DAYS

OTHER NOTES/COMMENTS: _____

_____

Total Payments (CCYY)

Indicate below the name of the insured and their dependents. When any of the following information is received, write it in pencil followed by the date. This will help you to realize when a patient's deductible has been met and if they are nearing any maximum benefit.

	INSURED	DEPENDENT	DEPENDENT	DEPENDENT	DEPENDENT
NAME:	_____	_____	_____	_____	_____
DEDUCTIBLE:	_____	_____	_____	_____	_____
COINS PD:	_____	_____	_____	_____	_____
LIFETIME:	_____	_____	_____	_____	_____

Appendix A

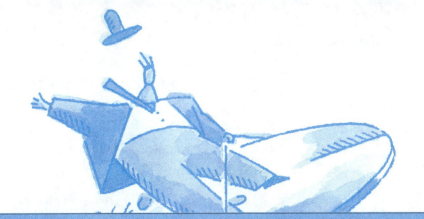

Table of Contents

Order of Benefit Determination

Rule #	Description
1	The plan without a COB provision will be primary to a plan with a COB provision.
2	When a plan does not have OBD rules, and as a result the plans do not agree on the OBD, the plan without these OBD rules will determine the order of payment.
3	The plan that covers an individual as an employee will be primary to a plan that covers that individual as a dependent.
4	If an individual is an employee under two plans, the primary is the one under which the employee has been covered the longest.
5	If an employee is an active employee under one plan and a retiree (or laid off) under another, the active plan will pay as primary.
The parent birthday rule, explained in #6 and #7, affects the OBD for dependent children of parents who are living together and married (not divorced or legally separated).	
6	The plan of the parent whose birthday (based on month and day only) occurs first during the calendar year is the primary plan.
7	When both parents' birthdays are the same (based on month and day), the benefits of the plan that covered one parent the longest is the primary plan.
For dependents of legally separated or divorced parents and those whose parents have remarried, the order of benefits determination is based on the following rule:	
8	The plan of the parent specified as having legal responsibility for the health-care expense of the child is the primary plan.
For dependents of separated parents with no court decree:	
9	The plan of the parent with custody is prime.
10	The plan of the step-parent (if any) with whom the child resides is secondary.
11	The plan of the natural parent without custody is tertiary.
12	The step-parent (if any) who does not reside with the child has no legal right to declare dependency. Therefore, no coordination should be performed because the child is probably not an eligible dependent under the plan.
13	For joint custody, with no additional responsibility designation, the plan of the parent whose coverage has been in effect the longest would be the primary payer. However, this rule may vary by administrator. Some parents pay costs on a 50/50 basis, thereby sharing equally in the health care risk.

■ **Table AA–1** Order of Benefit Determination

Medicare Secondary Payer

If the patient...	And this condition exists...	Then the program pays first...	And this program pays second...
Is age 65 or older, and is covered by a Group Health Plan through a current employer or spouse's current employer...	The employer has less than 20 employees...	**Medicare**	Group Health Plan
	The employer has 20 or more employees, or at least one employer is a multiemployer group that employs 20 or more individuals...	Group Health Plan	**Medicare**
Has an employer retirement plan and is age 65 or older or is disabled and age 65 or older...	The patient is entitled to Medicare...	**Medicare**	Retiree coverage
Is disabled and covered by a Large Group Health Plan from work, or is covered by a family member who is working...	The employer has less than 100 employees...	**Medicare**	Large Group Health Plan
	The employer has 100 or more employees, or at least one employer is a multiemployer group that employs 100 or more individuals...	Large Group Health Plan	**Medicare**
Has end-stage renal disease and Group Health Plan Coverage...	Is in the first 30 months of eligibility or entitlement to Medicare...	Group Health Plan	**Medicare**
	After 30 months...	**Medicare**	Group Health Plan
Has end-stage renal disease and COBRA coverage...	Is in the first 30 months of eligibility or entitlement to Medicare...	COBRA	Medicare
	After 30 months...	**Medicare**	COBRA
Is covered under workers' compensation because of job-related illness or injury...	The patient is entitled to Medicare...	Workers' compensation (for health-care items or services related to job-related illness or injury)	**Medicare**
Has black lung disease and is covered under the Federal Black Lung Program...	The patient is eligible for the Federal Black Lung Program...	Federal Black Lung Program (for health-care services related to black lung disease)	**Medicare**
Has been in an auto accident where no-fault or liability insurance is involved...	The patient is entitled to Medicare...	No-fault or liability insurance (for accident-related health-care services)	**Medicare**
Is age 65 or older OR is disabled and covered by Medicare and COBRA...	The patient is entitled to Medicare...	**Medicare**	COBRA
Has Veterans Health Administration (VHA) benefits...	Receives VHA authorized health care services at a non-VHA facility...	VHA	Medicare may pay when the services provided are Medicare-covered services and are not covered by the VHA

■ **Table AA–2** Medicare Secondary Payer

Quick Reference Codes

ORGANIZATION OF VOLUME I	
Number	**Body System/Classification**
00–13	Infective and Parasitic Diseases
14–23	Neoplasms
24–27	Endocrine, Nutritional, Metabolic Diseases
28	Diseases of the Blood and Blood-Forming Organs
29–31	Mental/Nervous Disorders
32–38	Diseases of the Nervous System and Sense Organs
39–45	Diseases of the Circulatory System
46–51	Diseases of the Respiratory System
52–57	Diseases of the Digestive System
58–62	Diseases of the Genito-Urinary System
63–67	Complications of Pregnancy, Childbirth and the Puerperium
68–70	Diseases of the Skin and Subcutaneous Tissue
71–73	Diseases of the Musculoskeletal System and Connective Tissue
74–75	Congenital Anomalies
76–77	Certain Causes of Perinatal Morbidity and Mortality
78–79	Symptoms, Signs and Ill-Defined Conditions
80–86	Fractures, Dislocations, Sprains and Internal Injuries
87–90	Lacerations
91–99	Other Accidents, Poisoning and Violence (nature of the injury)
V0–Y24	Miscellaneous Informative Codings (a particular diagnosis is not indicated)

SECTIONS OF THE CPT®AND RVS	
Code	**Description**
99201–99499	**Evaluation and Management**
CPT®00100–01999 RVS 10000–69999 99100–99140	**Anesthesia:**
10021–69999	**Surgery**
70010–79999	**Radiology/Nuclear Medicine**
80048–89356	**Pathology and Laboratory Tests**
90281–99199 and 99500–99602	**Medicine**

EVALUATION AND MANAGEMENT CODES	
Code	**Description**
99201–99215	Office or Other Outpatient Services
99217–99220	Hospital Observation Services
99221–99239	Hospital Inpatient Services
99241–99275	Consultations
99281–99288	Emergency Department Services
99289–99290	Pediatric Critical Care Patient Transport
99291–99292	Critical Care Services
99293–99296	Inpatient Neonatal and Pediatric Critical Care Services
99298–99299	Intensive (Noncritical) Low-Birth-Weight Services
99301–99316	Nursing Facility Services
99321–99333	Domiciliary, Rest Home, or Custodial Care Services
99341–99350	Home Services

■ **Table AA–3** Quick Reference Codes

(continues on next page)

99354–99360	Prolonged Services
99361–99373	Case Management Services
99374–99380	Care Plan Oversite Services
99381–99429	Preventive Medicine Services
99431–99440	Newborn Care Services
99450–9945	Special Evaluation and Management Services
99499	Other Evaluation and Management Services

ANESTHESIA CODES

Code	Description
00100–00222	Head
00300–00352	Neck
00400–00474	Thorax
00500–00580	Intrathoracic
00600–00670	Spine and Spinal Cord
00700–00797	Upper Abdomen
00800–00882	Lower Abdomen
00902–00952	Perineum
01112–01190	Pelvis (Except Hip)
01200–01274	Upper Leg (Except Knee)
01320–01444	Knee and Popliteal Area
01420–01522	Lower Leg
01710–01782	Upper Arm and Elbow
01810–01860	Forearm, Wrist and Hand
01905–01933	Radiological Procedures
01951–01953	Burns, Excisions or Debridement
01958–01969	Obstetric
01990–01999	Other Procedures

SURGERY CODES

Code	Description
10040–19499	Integumentary System
20000–29999	Musculoskeletal System
30000–32999	Respiratory System
33010–37799	Cardiovascular System
38100–38999	Hemic and Lymphatic System
39000–39599	Mediastinum and Diaphragm
40490–49999	Digestive System
50010–53899	Urinary System
54000–55899	Male Genital System
55970–55980	Intersex Surgery
56400–58999	Female Genital System
59000–59899	Maternity Care and Delivery
60000–60699	Endocrine System
61000–64999	Nervous System
65091–68899	Eye and Ocular Adnexa
69000–69979	Auditory System
69990	Operating Microscope
93501–93553	Cardiac Catheterizations

(continues on next page)

RADIOLOGY CODES

Code	Description
70010–76499	Diagnostic Radiology
76506–76999	Diagnostic Ultrasound
77261–77799	Radiation Oncology
78000–79999	Nuclear Medicine

PATHOLOGY CODES

Code	Description
80048–80076	Organ or Disease Oriented Panels
80100–80103	Drug Testing
80150–80299	Therapeutic Drug Assays
80400–80440	Evocative/Suppression Testing
80500–80502	Consultations (Clinical Pathology)
81000–81099	Urinalysis
82000–84999	Chemistry
85002–85999	Hematology and Coagulation
86000–86849	Immunology
86850–86999	Transfusion Medicine
87001–87999	Microbiology
88000–88099	Anatomic Pathology
88104–88199	Cytopathology
88230–88299	Cytogenic Studies
88300–88399	Surgical Pathology
88400	Transcutaneous Procedures
89050–89240	Other Procedures
89250–89356	Reproductive Medicine Procedures

MEDICINE CODES

Code	Description
90281–90399	Immune Globulins
90471–90474	Immunization Administration for Vaccines/Toxoids
90476–90749	Vaccines/Toxoids
90780–90781	Therapeutic or Diagnostic Infusions
90782–90799	Therapeutic, Prophylactic or Diagnostic Injections
90801–90899	Psychiatry
90900–90911	Biofeedback
90918–90999	Dialysis
91000–91299	Gastroenterology
92002–92499	Ophthalmology
92502–92700	Special Otorhinolaryngologic Services
92950–93799	Cardiovascular
93875–93990	Noninvasive Vascular Studies
94010–94799	Pulmonary
95004–95199	Allergy and Clinical Immunology
95250	Endocrinology
95805–96004	Neurology and Neuromuscular Procedures
96100–96117	Central Nervous System Assessments/Tests
96150–96155	Health and Behavior Assessment /Intervention

(continues on next page)

96400–96549	Chemotherapy Administration
96567–96571	Photodynamic Therapy
96900–96999	Special Dermatological Procedures
97001–97799	Physical Medicine and Rehabilitation
97802–97804	Medical Nutrition Therapy
97810–97814	Acupuncture
98925–98929	Osteopathic Manipulative Treatment
98940–98943	Chiropractic Manipulative Treatment
99000–99091	Special Services, Procedures and Reports

Place of Service Codes

Place of Service	Description
01	**Pharmacy** (A facility or location where drugs and other medically related items and services are sold, dispensed, or otherwise provider directly to patients.)
02	**Unassigned** N/A
03	**School** (A facility whose primary purpose is education.)
04	**Homeless Shelter** (A facility or location whose primary purpose is to provide temporary housing to homeless individuals (e.g., emergency shelters, individual or family shelters.)
05	**Indian Health Service Free-standing** (A facility or location, owned and operated by the Indian Health Service, which provides diagnostic, therapeutic (surgical and nonsurgical), and rehabilitation services to American Indians and Alaska Natives who do not require hospitalization.)
06	**Indian Health Service Provider-based Facility** (A facility or location, owned and operated by the Indian Health Service, which provides diagnostic, therapeutic (surgical and nonsurgical), and rehabilitation services rendered by, or under the supervision of, physicians to American Indians and Alaska Natives admitted as inpatients or outpatients.)
07	**Tribal 638 Free-standing Facility** (A facility or location owned and operated by a federally recognized American Indian or Alaska Native tribe or tribal organization under a 638 agreement, which provides diagnostic, therapeutic (surgical and nonsurgical), and rehabilitation services to tribal members who do not require hospitalization.)
08	**Tribal 638 Provider-based Facility** (A facility or location owned and operated by a federally recognized American Indian or Alaska Native tribe or tribal organization under a 638 agreement, which provides diagnostic, therapeutic (surgical and nonsurgical), and rehabilitation services to tribal members.)
09–10	**Unassigned** (N/A).
11	**Office** (Location other than a hospital, Skilled Nursing Facility [SNF], Military Treatment Facility, Community Health Center, State or Local Public Health Clinic or Intermediate Care Facility [ICF], where the health professional routinely provides health examinations, diagnosis, and treatment of illness or injury on an ambulatory basis.)
12	**Home** (Location other than a hospital or other facility where the patient received care in a private residence).
13	**Assisted Living Facility** (Congregate residential facility with self-contained living units providing assessment of each resident's needs and on-site support 24 hours a day, 7 days a week, with the capacity to deliver or arrange for services including some health care and other services.)
14	**Group Home (nonfacility)** (Congregate residential foster care setting for children and adolescents in state custody that provides some social, health-care, and educational support services and that promotes rehabilitation and reintegration of residents into the community).
15	**Mobile Unit** (A facility/unit that moves from place-to-place equipped to provide preventive, screening, diagnostic, and/or treatment services.)
16–19	**Unassigned**
20	**Urgent Care Facility** (Location, distinct from a hospital emergency room, an office, or a clinic, whose purpose is to diagnose and treat illness or injury for unscheduled, ambulatory patients seeking immediate medical attention.)
21	**Inpatient Hospital** (A facility other than psychiatric, which primarily provides diagnostic, therapeutic (both surgical and nonsurgical) and rehabilitation services by, or under the supervision of, physicians to patients admitted for a variety of medical conditions.)
22	**Outpatient Hospital** (A portion of a hospital that provides diagnostic, therapeutic (both surgical and nonsurgical) and rehabilitation services to sick and injured persons who do not require hospitalization or institutionalization.) A patient who is not admitted to a hospital (i.e., one who is under 24-hour supervision) is an outpatient.
23	**Emergency Room—Hospital** (A portion of a hospital where emergency diagnosis and treatment of illness or injury is provided.) Patients in the emergency room are considered to be facility outpatients. (Remember to also complete box 24I.)

■ **Table AA–4** Place of Service Codes

(continues on next page)

24	**Ambulatory Surgical Center (ASC)** (A freestanding facility other than a physician's office where surgical and diagnostic services are provided on an ambulatory basis.) When this code is used, the facility must be a CMS-approved ASC.
25	**Birthing Center** (A facility other than a hospital's maternity facilities or a physician's office that provides a setting for labor, delivery, and immediate postpartum care as well as immediate care of newborn infants.)
26	**Military Treatment Facility** (MTF) (A medical facility operated by one or more of the Uniformed Services. MTF also refers to certain former U.S. Public Health Service facilities now designated as Uniformed Service Treatment Facilities (USTF).)
27–30	**Unassigned**
31	**Skilled Nursing Facility** (A facility that primarily provides inpatient skilled nursing care and related services to patients who require medical, nursing, or rehabilitative services and does not provide the level of care or treatment available in a hospital.)
32	**Nursing Facility** (A facility that provides skilled nursing care and related services for the rehabilitation of injured, disabled, or sick persons or on a regular basis health-related care services above the level of custodial care to other than mentally retarded individuals.)
33	**Custodial Care Facility** (A facility that provides room, board and personal assistance services, generally on a long-term basis, and that does not include a medical component.)
34	**Hospice** (A facility, other than a patient's home, in which palliative and supportive care for terminally ill patients and their families is provided.)
35–40	**Unassigned**
41	**Ambulance—Land** (A land vehicle specifically designed, equipped and staffed for lifesaving and transporting the sick or injured.)
42	**Ambulance—Air or Water** (An air or water vehicle specifically designed, equipped and staffed for lifesaving and transporting the sick or injured.)
43–48	**Unassigned**
49	**Independent Clinic (nonfacility)** (A location, not part of a hospital and not described by any other Place of Service code, that is organized and operated to provide preventive, diagnostic, therapeutic, rehabilitative, or palliative services to outpatients only.)
50	**Federally Qualified Health Center** (A facility located in a medically underserved area that provides Medicare beneficiaries preventive primary medical care under the general direction of a physician.)
51	**Inpatient Psychiatric Facility** (A facility that provides inpatient psychiatric services for the diagnosis and treatment of mental illness on a 24-hour basis, by or under the supervision of a physician.)
52	**Psychiatric Facility-Partial Hospitalization** (A facility for the diagnosis and treatment of mental illness that provides a planned therapeutic program for patients who do not need full-time hospitalization, but who need broader programs than are possible from outpatient visits in a hospital-based or hospital-affiliated facility.)
53	**Community Mental Health Center** (A facility that provides comprehensive mental health services on an ambulatory basis, primarily to individuals residing or employed in a defined area. Includes a physician-directed mental health facility.)
54	**Intermediate Care Facility/Mentally Retarded** (A facility that primarily provides health-related care and services above the level of custodial care of mentally retarded individuals but does not provide the level of care or treatment available in a hospital or SNF.)
55	**Residential Substance Abuse Treatment Facility** (A facility that provides treatment for substance (alcohol and drug) abuse to live-in residents who do not require acute medical care. Services include individual and group therapy and counseling, family counseling, laboratory tests, drugs and supplies, psychological testing, and room and board.)
56	**Psychiatric Residential Treatment Center** (A facility or distinct part of a facility for psychiatric care that provides a total 24-hour therapeutically planned and professionally staffed group living and learning environment.)
57	**Nonresidential Substance Abuse Treatment Facility (nonfacility)** (A location that provides treatment for substance (alcohol and drug) abuse on an ambulatory basis. Services include individual and group therapy and counseling, family counseling, laboratory tests, drugs and supplies, and psychological testing.)

(continues on next page)

58–59	Unassigned
60	**Mass Immunization Center** (A location where providers administer pneumococcal pneumonia and influenza virus vaccinations and submit these services as electronic media claims, paper claims, or using the roster billing method. This generally takes place in a mass immunization setting, such as a public health center, pharmacy, or mall, but may include a physician office setting.)
61	**Comprehensive Inpatient Rehabilitation Facility** (A facility that provides comprehensive rehabilitation services under the supervision of a physician to inpatients with physical disabilities. Services include rehabilitation nursing, physical therapy, occupational therapy, speech pathology, social or psychological services, and orthotics and prosthetics services. There are specific licensing requirements for these facilities.)
62	**Comprehensive Outpatient Rehabilitation Facility** (A facility that provides comprehensive rehabilitation services under the supervision of a physician to inpatients with physical disabilities. Services include physical therapy, occupational therapy, and speech pathology services. There are specific licensing requirements for these facilities.)
63–64	Unassigned
65	**End Stage Renal Disease Treatment Facility** (A facility other than a hospital, that provides dialysis treatment, maintenance, and/or training to patients or caregivers on an ambulatory or home-care basis.)
66–70	Unassigned
71	**State or Local Public Health Clinic** (A facility maintained by either state or local health departments that provides ambulatory primary medical care under the general direction of a physician. Such facilities must be physician-directed.)
72	**Rural Health Clinic** (A certified facility that is located in a rural medically underserved area that provides ambulatory primary medical care under the general direction of a physician. Qualified facilities do not bill Part B of Medicare for items or services except for DME and orthotics and prosthetics.)
73–80	Unassigned
81	**Independent Laboratory** (A laboratory certified to perform diagnostic and/or clinical tests independent of an institution or a physician's office.) With the exception of hospital inpatients, the place of service for lab tests will be based on where "drawn" instead of where the test is actually performed. If the physician is billing for a lab service performed in his/her own office, then use the appropriate code for provider's office. If an independent laboratory is billing, show the place where the sample is drawn. An independent laboratory drawing a sample in its laboratory shows the code for independent laboratory as the place of service. If an independent laboratory is billing for a test on a sample drawn on a hospital inpatient, then the appropriate code for hospital inpatient is entered as the place of service. If the independent laboratory is billing for a test on a sample drawn in a physician's office, then the appropriate code is for provider's office.
82–98	Unassigned
99	**Other Unlisted Facility** (Other service facilities not identified above.)

State Abbreviations

NAME OF STATE	ABBREVIATION
Alabama	AL
Alaska	AK
American Samoa	AS
Arizona	AZ
Arkansas	AR
California	CA
Colorado	CO
Connecticut	CT
Delaware	DE
District of Columbia	DC
Florida	FL
Georgia	GA
Guam	GU
Hawaii	HI
Idaho	ID
Illinois	IL
Indiana	IN
Iowa	IA
Kansas	KS
Kentucky	KY
Louisiana	LA
Maine	ME
Maryland	MD
Massachusetts	MA
Michigan	MI
Minnesota	MN
Mississippi	MD
Missouri	MO
Montana	MT
Nebraska	NE
Nevada	NV
New Hampshire	NH
New Jersey	NJ
New Mexico	NM
New York	NY
North Carolina	NC
North Dakota	ND
Ohio	OH
Oklahoma	OK
Oregon	OR
Pennsylvania	PA
Puerto Rico	PR
Rhode Island	RI
South Carolina	SC
South Dakota	SD
Tennessee	TN
Texas	TX
Utah	UT
Vermont	VT

■ **Table AA–5** State Abbreviations   *(continues on next page)*

Virginia	VA
Virgin Islands	VI
Washington	WA
West Virginia	WV
Wisconsin	WI
Wyoming	WY

Other Address Abbreviations

OTHER ADDRESS	ABBREVIATION
Alley	Aly
Avenue	Ave
Boulevard	Blvd
Branch	Br
Bypass	Byp
Causeway	Cswy
Center	Ctr
Circle	Cir
Court	Ct
Courts	Cts
Crescent	Cres
Drive	Dr
Expressway	Expy
Extension	Ext
Freeway	Fwy
Gardens	Gdns
Grove	Grv
Heights	Hts
Highway	Hwy
Lane	Ln
Manor	Mnr
Place	Pl
Plaza	Plz
Point	Pt
Post Office	PO
Road	Rd
Rural	R
Rural Route	RR
Square	Sq
Street	St
Terrace	Ter
Trail	Trl
Turnpike	Tpke
Viaduct	Via
Vista	Vis

■ **Table AA–6** Other Address Abbreviations

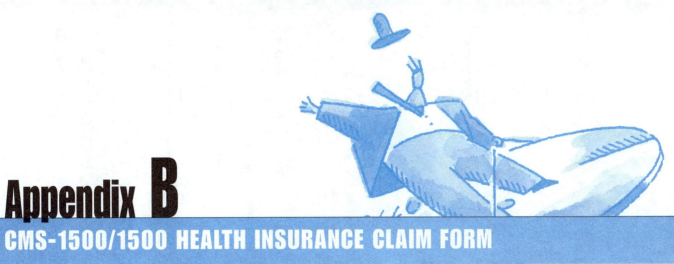

Appendix B

CMS-1500/1500 HEALTH INSURANCE CLAIM FORM

Table of Contents

Header—Top of Form   **Purpose: Directs the claim to the appropriate payer.**

1500
HEALTH INSURANCE CLAIM FORM
□□□ PICA   PICA □□□

← CARRIER →

Information to Enter	Commercial/Private	Medicare	Medicaid	Workers' Compensation
Enter the name and address of the payer(s) to whom this claim is being sent. Use spaces to separate names. Enter address information as follows: 1st line=Name; 2nd line=First line of address; 3rd line=Second line of address, if necessary; and 4th line=city, state (2 digits) and zip code. Do not use punctuation except "#" and "-." If an attention line is needed place it in the second line.	Required.	Required.	Required.	Required.

Block 1—Insurance Coverage Information   **Purpose: Shows the type of health insurance coverage applicable to this claim.**

1. MEDICARE   MEDICAID   TRICARE CHAMPUS   CHAMPVA   GROUP HEALTH PLAN   FECA BLKLUNG   OTHER

□ (Medicare #)   □ (Medicaid #)   □ (Sponsor's SSN)   □ (Member ID#)   ☒ (SSN or ID)   □ (SSN)   □ (ID)

Information to Enter	Commercial/Private	Medicare	Medicaid	Workers' Compensation
Enter an X in the applicable box.	For an Individual Plan place an X in "OTHER." For a Group Plan place an X in "GROUP."	Enter an X in the "MEDICARE" box.	Enter an X in the "MEDICAID" box.	Enter an X in "OTHER," unless diagnosis is for "FECA BLK LUNG." If FECA, place an X in that box.

Block 1a—Insured's Identification, Policy or Certificate Number and Group Number   **Purpose: Identifies the patient to the payer.**

1a INSURED'S I.D. NUMBER   (For Program in Item1)

Information to Enter	Commercial/Private	Medicare	Medicaid	Workers' Compensation
Enter the insured's identification number as shown on the insured's health	Required.	Enter the patient's	Enter the	Enter the patient's WC

(continues on next page)

■ **Table AB–1** 1500 Health Insurance Claim Form Matrix

insurance card for the payer to whom the claim is being submitted. Do not use punctuation.

| Medicare HICN. | patient's Medicaid ID number, complete with any prefixes and suffixes. | claim number if available. If not, enter employer's policy number, or patient's SSN. If a SSN is not available, a driver's license number and jurisdiction, a green card number, a visa number, or passport number can be used. |

Block 2—Patient's Name   Purpose: Identifies the patient.

2. PATIENT'S NAME (Last Name, First Name, Middle Initial).

Information to Enter	Commercial/Private	Medicare	Medicaid	Workers' Compensation
Enter the patient's full last name, first name, and middle initial. Use spaces to separate names. If the patient uses a last name suffix (i.e., Jr, Sr) enter it after the last name and before the first name. Do not use punctuation except a "-", which may be used for hyphenated names.	Required.	Required.	Required.	Required.

Block 3—Patient's Birth Date   Purpose: Identifies the patient; distinguishes persons with similar names.

3. PATIENT'S BIRTH DATE
MM DD YY   SEX
                  M ☐ F ☐

Information to Enter	Commercial/Private	Medicare	Medicaid	Workers' Compensation
Enter the patient's date of birth. Use the eight-digit numeric date (MM DD CCYY). Use spaces to separate parts of the field. Enter an X in the correct box to indicate the sex of the patient.	Required.	Required.	Required.	Required.

Block 4—Insured's Name   Purpose: Identifies the patient's source of insurance.

4. INSURED'S NAME (Last Name, First Name, Middle Initial)

Information to Enter	Commercial/Private	Medicare	Medicaid	Workers' Compensation
Enter the insured's full last name, first name, and middle initial. If the insured uses a last name suffix (i.e., Jr, Sr) enter it after the last name and before the first name. Use spaces to separate names. Do not use punctuation except a "-"; which may be used for hyphenated names. If the patient and insured are the same enter "SAME."	Required.	If Medicare is the primary carrier, leave empty. If not, list name.	If insured is also the patient, leave empty. If not, list name.	Enter the name of the patient's employer.

(continues on next page)

Block 5—Patient's Address   Purpose: Further identifies patient; allows contact for questions.

5. PATIENT'S ADDRESS (No., Street)

CITY | STATE

ZIP CODE | TELEPHONE (Include Area Code)
( )

Information to Enter

Enter the patient's mailing address and telephone number. Do not use punctuation except "#" and "-". Use the two-digit state code and if available nine-digit zip code.

Commercial/Private	Medicare	Medicaid	Workers' Compensation
Required.	Required.	Required.	Required.

Block 6—Patient's Relationship to Insured   Purpose: Identifies patient's source of insurance; also distinguishes patient from insured.

6. PATIENT'S RELATIONSHIP TO INSURED

Self ☐ Spouse ☐ Child ☐ Other ☐

Information to Enter

Enter an X in the correct box to indicate the patient's relationship to the insured. For unmarried domestic partner check the "OTHER" box.

Commercial/Private	Medicare	Medicaid	Workers' Compensation
Required.	Use only if block 4 is completed.	Leave empty, unless there is other coverage.	Enter an X in the "OTHER" box.

Block 7—Insured's Address   Purpose: Further identifies insured; allows contact for questions.

7. INSURED'S ADDRESS (No., Street)

CITY | STATE

ZIP CODE | TELEPHONE (Include Area Code)
( )

Information to Enter

Enter the insured's address and telephone number. Do not use punctuation except "#" and "-". Use the two-digit state code and if available nine-digit zip code. Enter "SAME" if block 4 is completed and the address is the same as block 5.

Commercial/Private	Medicare	Medicaid	Workers' Compensation
Required.	Complete only if block 4 is completed.	Complete only if block 4 is completed.	Enter the address and telephone number of the patient's employer.

(continues on next page)

Block 8—Patient Status   Purpose: Allows determination of liability and COB.

8. PATIENT STATUS

Single ☐	Married ☐	Other ☐
Employed ☐	Full-Time Student ☐	Part-Time Student ☐

Information to Enter	Commercial/Private	Medicare	Medicaid	Workers' Compensation
Enter an X in the box for the patient's marital status and for the patient's employment or student status. If widowed or divorced select the "Single" box. Use "Other" for domestic partner.	Required.	Required.	Not required.	Enter an X in the "Employed" box.

Block 9—Other Insured's Name   Purpose: Identifies other sources of insurance.

9. OTHER INSURED'S NAME (Last Name, First Name, Middle Initial)

Information to Enter	Commercial/Private	Medicare	Medicaid	Workers' Compensation
If item 11d is marked, complete fields 9–9-d, otherwise leave blank. Enter the name of the holder of a secondary or other policy that may cover the patient. Enter the other insured's full last name, first name, and middle initial of the enrollee in another health plan. Use spaces to separate names. Do not use punctuation except a "-"; which may be used for hyphenated names. If the patient and insured are the same enter "SAME."	Required.	If Medicare is the primary insurer leave 9–9d empty. If not, enter info.	If Medicaid is the primary insurer leave 9–9d empty. If not, enter info.	Not required unless claim has not been declared WC.

Block 9a—Other Insured's Policy or Group Number   Purpose: Identifies other sources of insurance.

a. OTHER INSURED'S POLICY OR GROUP NUMBER

Information to Enter	Commercial/Private	Medicare	Medicaid	Workers' Compensation
Enter the policy or group number of the other insured as indicated in block 9. Copy the number from the health identification card. Complete only if block 9 is completed.	Required.	Indicate "Medigap" if Medigap insurance is listed.	Required.	Not required unless claim has not been declared WC.

(continues on next page)

Block 9b—Other Insured's Date of Birth — Purpose: Identifies other insurance source. Also used to determine the primary source of insurance.

b. OTHER INSURED'S DATE OF BIRTH
MM | DD | YY   SEX M ☐ F ☐

Information to Enter	Commercial/Private	Medicare	Medicaid	Workers' Compensation
Enter the date of birth and sex of the other insured as indicated in block 9. Enter an X in the correct box to indicate the sex of the other insured. Use the eight-digit numeric date (MM DD CCYY). Use spaces to separate parts of the field. Complete only if block 9 is completed.	Required.	Required.	Required.	Not required unless claim has not been declared WC.

Block 9c—Employer's Name or School Name — Purpose: Identifies other sources of insurance.

c. EMPLOYER'S NAME OR SCHOOL NAME

Information to Enter	Commercial/Private	Medicare	Medicaid	Workers' Compensation
Enter the name of the other insured's employer or school as indicated in block 9. Complete only if block 9 completed.	Required.	Required.	Required.	Not required unless claim has not been declared WC.

Block 9d—Insurance Plan Name or Program Name — Purpose: Identifies other sources of insurance.

d. INSURANCE PLAN NAME OR PROGRAM NAME

Information to Enter	Commercial/Private	Medicare	Medicaid	Workers' Compensation
Enter the other insured's insurance plan or program name. Complete only if block 9 completed.	Required.	Required.	Required.	Not required unless claim has not been declared WC.

Block 10a–10c—Is Patient's Condition Related to Employment? — Purpose: Identifies primary liability for condition.

10. IS PATIENT'S CONDITION RELATED TO:

a. EMPLOYMENT? (Current or Previous)
☐ YES ☐ NO

b. AUTO ACCIDENT?   PLACE (State)
☐ YES ☐ NO ____

c. OTHER ACCIDENT?
☐ YES ☐ NO

Information to Enter	Commercial/Private	Medicare	Medicaid	Workers' Compensation

(continues on next page)

	Commercial/Private	Medicare	Medicaid	Workers' Compensation
Enter an X in the correct box to indicate whether one or more of the services described in Item 24 are for a condition or injury that occurred on-the-job or as a result of an automobile or other accident. The state postal code must be shown if "YES" is checked in 10b for "Auto Accident." Any item marked "Yes" indicates that there may be other applicable insurance coverage that would be primary, such as automobile liability insurance.	Required.	Enter an X in the "No" box. If "Yes," the other payer should be billed as primary, before billing Medicare.	Enter an X in the "No" box. If "Yes," the other payer should be billed as primary, before billing Medicaid.	Enter an X in the "Yes" box for 10a.

Block 10d—Reserved for Local Use?   Purpose: To be determined by local payer.

10d.   RESERVED FOR LOCAL USE

Information to Enter	Commercial/Private	Medicare	Medicaid	Workers' Compensation
Refer to the most current instructions from the applicable public or private payer regarding the use of this field.	Per payer specifications; otherwise leave empty.	Per payer specifications; otherwise leave empty.	Per payer specifications; otherwise leave empty.	Per payer specifications; otherwise leave empty.

Block 11—Insured's Policy Group or FECA Number   Purpose: Identifies insured's policy or group number.

11.   INSURED'S POLICY GROUP OR FECA NUMBER

Information to Enter	Commercial/Private	Medicare	Medicaid	Workers' Compensation
Enter the insured's policy or group number as it appears on the insured's health care identification card. The FECA number is a 9-digit alphanumeric identifier assigned to a patient claiming work-related conditions under FECA.	Required.	If Medicare is the primary insurance carrier, list "NONE" and proceed to block 12. If there is a terminating event with regard to insurance (e.g., insured retired) enter "NONE" and proceed to block 11b.	Not required.	Not required.

Block 11a—Insured's Date of Birth   Purpose: Identifies other sources of insurance. Used to determine the primary source of insurance.

a. INSURED'S DATE OF BIRTH
MM   DD   YY   SEX   M ☐   F ☐

(continues on next page)

Information to Enter	Commercial/Private	Medicare	Medicaid	Workers' Compensation
Enter the insured's date of birth (this refers to the insured indicated in block 1a). Enter an X in the correct box to indicate the sex of the insured. Use the eight-digit numeric date (MM DD CCYY). Use spaces to separate parts of the field.	Required.	Not required.	Not required.	Not required.

Block 11b—Employer's Name or School Name   Purpose: Identifies other sources of insurance.

b. EMPLOYER'S NAME OR SCHOOL NAME

Information to Enter	Commercial/Private	Medicare	Medicaid	Workers' Compensation
Enter the name of the insured's employer or school.	Required.	If a change in the insured's insurance status has occurred enter the reason (e.g., RETIRED).	Not required.	Not required.

Block 11c—Insurance Plan Name or Program Name   Purpose: Identifies other sources of insurance.

c. INSURANCE PLAN NAME OR PROGRAM NAME

Information to Enter	Commercial/Private	Medicare	Medicaid	Workers' Compensation
Enter the insured's insurance plan or program name.	Required.	Not Required.	Not required.	Not required.

Block 11d—Is There Another Health Benefit Plan?   Purpose: Identifies other sources of insurance.

d. IS THERE ANOTHER HEALTH BENEFIT PLAN?

☐ YES ☐ NO   *If yes, return to and complete item 9 a–d*

Information to Enter	Commercial/Private	Medicare	Medicaid	Workers' Compensation
When appropriate enter an X in the correct box, if there is another health benefit plan other than the plan indicated in block 1. If marked "YES" complete blocks 9–9d.	Required.	Required.	Required.	Not required, unless claim has not been declared WC, then enter an X in the "Yes" box and complete 9–9d.

(continues on next page)

224

Block 12—Authorization for Release of Medical Information   Purpose: Gives permission to release any medical or other information necessary to process and/or adjudicate the claim.

READ BACK OF FORM BEFORE COMPLETING & SIGNING THIS FORM

12. PATIENT'S OR AUTHORIZED PERSON'S SIGNATURE I authorize the release of any medical or other information necessary to process this claim. I also request payment of government benefits either to myself or to the party who accepts assignment below.

SIGNED _____ DATE _____

Information to Enter	Commercial/Private	Medicare	Medicaid	Workers' Compensation
Enter "Signature on File", "SOF" or legal signature. When a legal signature is provided, enter date signed in the six-digit format (MMDDYY) or eight-digit (MMDDCCYY) format. If there is no signature on file, leave blank or enter "No Signature on File."	Required.	Required.	Not required.	Not required.

Block 13—Authorization for Assignment of Benefits to Provider   Purpose: Gives permission authorizing payment of benefits to the provider of services.

13. INSURED'S OR AUTHORIZED PERSON'S SIGNATURE I authorize payment of medical benefits to the undersigned physician or supplier for services described below.

SIGNED _____

Information to Enter	Commercial/Private	Medicare	Medicaid	Workers' Compensation
Enter "Signature on File", "SOF" or legal signature. If there is no signature on file, leave blank or enter "No Signature on File."	Required.	Required.	Not required.	Not required.

Block 14—Date of Illness, Injury, or Pregnancy   Purpose: Helps payers identify benefits.

14. DATE OF CURRENT: ILLNESS (First symptom) OR
MM   DD   YY   ◄ INJURY (Accident) OR
         PREGNANCY (LMP)

Information to Enter	Commercial/Private	Medicare	Medicaid	Workers' Compensation
Enter the first date of the present illness, injury, or pregnancy. Use the six-digit format (MM DD YY). Use spaces to separate parts of the field. For pregnancy, use the date of the last menstrual period.	Required.	Required.	Not required.	Requires a specific date for the on-the-job illness or injury. The date should be the same as that indicated on the Doctor's First Report.

(continues on next page)

Block 15—If Patient Has Had Same or Similar Illness, Give First Date   Purpose: Allows determination of liability and COB.

15. IF PATIENT HAS HAD SAME OR SIMILAR ILLNESS,
    GIVE FIRST DATE   MM │ DD │ YY

Information to Enter	Commercial/Private	Medicare	Medicaid	Workers' Compensation
Enter the first date that the patient had the same or a similar illness. Use the six-digit numeric date (MM DD YY). Use spaces to separate parts of the field.	Required.	Not required.	Not required.	Not required.

Block 16—Patient Disability Dates for Current Occupation   Purpose: Identifies dates of disability.

16. DATES PATIENT UNABLE TO WORK IN CURRENT OCCUPATION
    MM │ DD │ YY   MM │ DD │ YY
    FROM   TO

Information to Enter	Commercial/Private	Medicare	Medicaid	Workers' Compensation
If the patient is employed and is unable to work in current occupation, an eight-digit numeric date (MMDDCCYY) must be shown for the "from-to" dates that the patient is unable to work. An entry in this field may indicate employment-related insurance coverage.	Required.	Required.	Not required.	Required.

Block 17—Name of Referring Physician or Other Source   Purpose: Identifies referral source.

17. NAME OF REFERRING PHYSICIAN OR OTHER SOURCE

Information to Enter	Commercial/Private	Medicare	Medicaid	Workers' Compensation
Enter the name (First Name, Middle Initial, Last Name) and credentials of the professional who referred or ordered the service(s) or supply(s) on the claim. Use spaces to separate names. Do not use punctuation except a "-" which may be used for hyphenated names. For services billed by an assistant surgeon or anesthesiologist enter the name and credential of the primary surgeon. For DME claims enter the name of the prescribing provider.	Required.	Required.	Required.	Enter the SSN or EIN of the employer.

(continues on next page)

Block 17a—I.D. Number of Referring Physician   Purpose: Identifies referral source.

17a.
17b. NPI

Information to Enter	Commercial/Private	Medicare	Medicaid	Workers' Compensation
Enter the identifying number (i.e., NPI, UPIN, MHCP ID numbers) of the referring or ordering physician, or other source. Required when block 17 is completed.	Enter a UPIN, PIN or NPI number.	Enter a UPIN, PIN or NPI number.	Enter a UPIN, PIN or NPI number.	Enter a SSN or EIN number.

Block 18—Hospitalization Dates   Purpose: Identifies services related to an inpatient stay.

18. HOSPITALIZATION DATES RELATED TO CURRENT SERVICES
MM   DD   YY   MM   DD   YY
FROM   TO

Information to Enter	Commercial/Private	Medicare	Medicaid	Workers' Compensation
Enter the inpatient hospital admission date followed by the discharge date (if discharge has occurred). If not discharged, leave discharge date blank. Use the eight-digit numeric date (MM DD CCYY). Use spaces to separate parts of the field. This date is when a medical service is furnished as a result of, or subsequent to, a related hospitalization.	Required.	Required.	Required.	Required.

Block 19—Reserved for Local Use   Purpose: Provides additional information.

19. RESERVED FOR LOCAL USE

Information to Enter	Commercial/Private	Medicare	Medicaid	Workers' Compensation
Refer to the most current instructions from the applicable public or private payer regarding the use of this field.	Per payer specifications; otherwise leave empty.	Per payer specifications; otherwise leave empty.	Per payer specifications; otherwise leave empty.	Per payer specifications; otherwise leave empty.

Block 20—Outside Lab? $Charges   Purpose: Identifies purchased laboratory, pathology, or radiology services.

20. OUTSIDE LAB? $ CHARGES
☐ YES   ☐ NO

Information to Enter	Commercial/Private	Medicare	Medicaid	Workers' Compensation
Complete this field when billing for purchased services. Enter an X in the "Yes" box if the reported service(s) were performed by an outside laboratory. If "Yes", enter the purchase price. Do not use a dollar sign. Use	Required.	Required.	Enter an X in the "No" box as outside	Required.

(continues on next page)

227

a space to divide the dollars and cents. Enter an X in the "No" box if outside laboratory services(s) are not included on the claim. When "YES" is marked, enter the independent provider's name and address in Block 32.

laboratories must bill Medicaid directly.

Block 21—Diagnosis or Nature of Illness or Injury   Purpose: Supports the reason for the service(s) and provides information necessary to process the claim. The diagnosis must relate to the service(s) performed.

21. DIAGNOSIS OR NATURE OF ILLNESS OR INJURY. (Relate Items 1,2,3, or 4 to Item 24E by Line)

1. _____ . _____
2. _____ . _____
3. _____ . _____
4. _____ . _____

Commercial/Private	Medicare	Medicaid	Workers' Compensation
Required.	Required.	Required.	Required.

Information to Enter

Enter the patient's diagnosis/condition. Enter up to four ICD-9CM diagnosis codes. Relate lines 1,2,3,4 to the lines of service in 24E by line number. Use the highest level of specificity. Do not use punctuation.

Block 22—Medicaid Resubmission   Purpose: Use to identify a resubmission of an incorrectly processed Medicaid claim.

22. MEDICAID RESUBMISSION CODE   ORIGINAL REF. NO.

Commercial/Private	Medicare	Medicaid	Workers' Compensation
Not required.	Not required.	Enter the correct Medicaid Transaction Control Number.	Not required.

Information to Enter

List the original reference number for resubmitted claims. Refer to the most current instructions from the applicable public or private payer regarding the use of this field. Leave empty for all payers except Medicaid.

Block 23—Prior Authorization Number   Purpose: Determines eligibility of the current service(s).

23. PRIOR AUTHORIZATION NUMBER

Commercial/Private	Medicare	Medicaid	Workers' Compensation
Required.	Required.	Required.	Not required.

Information to Enter

Enter any of the following: prior authorization or pre-certification number; referral number; or CLIA number; as assigned by the payer for the current service when applicable. Notations such as "Prescription on File" can be noted for DME or pharmacy claims; or "SSO Performed" can be noted for claims which require an SSO to be performed.

(continues on next page)

Block 24A—Date(s) of Service [lines 1–6]   Purpose: Informs the payer of the date(s) of service(s).

24.	A				
	DATE(S) OF SERVICE				
	From		To		
MM	DD	YY	MM	DD	YY

Information to Enter	Commercial/Private	Medicare	Medicaid	Workers' Compensation
Enter date(s) of service, from and to: If one date of service only, enter the date under "From." Leave "To" blank or re-enter "From" date. If grouping services, the place of service, type of service, procedure code, charges and individual provider for each line must be identical for that service line. The number of days must correspond to the number of units in 24G. Use the six-digit numeric date (MM DD YY). Use spaces to separate parts of the field.	Required.	Required.	Leave "To" date empty. No date Ranging allowed.	Required.

Block 24B—Place of Service [lines 1–6]   Purpose: Informs the payer as to where the service(s) were performed.

B
PLACE
OF
SERVICE

Information to Enter	Commercial/Private	Medicare	Medicaid	Workers' Compensation
Enter the two-digit code for the "Place of Service" for each item used or service performed. Refer to the Place of Service list in Appendix C.	Required.	Required.	Required.	Required.

(continues on next page)

Block 24C—EMG [lines 1–6]   Purpose: Indicates if services were for emergency treatment in a hospital.

C
EMG

Information to Enter	Commercial/Private	Medicare	Medicaid	Workers' Compensation
If the provider does not have an NPI number, enter the appropriate qualifier and identifying number in the shaded area.	Per payer specifications; otherwise leave empty.	Per payer specifications; otherwise leave empty.	Per payer specifications; otherwise leave empty.	Not required.

Block 24D—Procedures, Services, or Supplies [lines 1–6]   Purpose: Informs payer as to what services were performed.

D
PROCEDURES, SERVICES, OR SUPPLIES
(Explain Unusual Circumstances)
CPT/HCPS   MODIFIER

Information to Enter	Commercial/Private	Medicare	Medicaid	Workers' Compensation
Enter the CPT® or HCPCS codes and modifier(s) (if applicable) from the appropriate code set in effect on the date of service. Use spaces to separate parts of field. Do not use hyphens for modifiers.	Required.	Required.	Required.	Required.

Block 24E—Diagnosis Code [lines 1–6]   Purpose: Informs the payer which diagnosis relates to each procedure.

E
DIAGNOSIS
POINTER

(continues on next page)

Information to Enter	Commercial/Private	Medicare	Medicaid	Workers' Compensation
Enter the diagnosis code reference number as shown in block 21 to relate the date of service and the procedures performed to the primary diagnosis. When multiple services are performed, the primary reference number for each service should be listed first, other applicable services should follow. The reference number(s) should be 1, or a 2, or a 3, or a 4; or multiple numbers as applicable. Do not use punctuation or enter ICD-9 codes here. Use spaces to separate line numbers.	Required.	Required.	Required.	Required.

Block 24F—$ Charges [lines 1–6]   Purpose: Informs the payer of the total amount charged for each service line.

F
$ CHARGES

Information to Enter	Commercial/Private	Medicare	Medicaid	Workers' Compensation
Enter the charge for each listed service. Enter numbers right justified in the dollar area of the field. If more than one date or unit is shown in 24G, the dollars shown should reflect the total of the services. Do not use dollar signs. Do not use commas as thousands marker. Use a space to separate parts of field.	Required.	Required.	Required.	Required.

Block 24G—Days or Units [lines 1–6]   Purpose: Informs the payer of the number or quantity of each service provided.

G
DAYS
OR
UNITS

231

(continues on next page)

Information to Enter	Commercial/Private	Medicare	Medicaid	Workers' Compensation
Enter the number of days or units for each service line. This field is most commonly used for multiple visits, units of supplies, anesthesia units or minutes, or oxygen volume. If only one service is performed, the number 1 must be entered. For anesthesia, enter the total minutes of anesthesia provided (convert hours to minutes).	Required.	Required.	Required.	Required.

Block 24H—EPSDT / Family Plan [lines 1–6]   Purpose: Indicates whether the services were for Early, Periodic, Screening, Diagnosis and Treatment services.

H						
EPSDT Family Plan						

Information to Enter	Commercial/Private	Medicare	Medicaid	Workers' Compensation
Leave empty unless Medicaid Claim.	Not required.	Not required.	Enter "E" for EPSDT services, or enter "F" for family planning services.	Not required.

Block 24I—EMG [lines 1–6]   Purpose: Indicates if services were for emergency treatment in a hospital.

I ID QUAL
NPI
NPI
NPI
NPI
NPI
NPI

(continues on next page)

Information to Enter	Commercial/Private	Medicare	Medicaid	Workers' Compensation
Check with payer to determine if this field is required. If required, enter Y for "YES" of leave blank if "NO"	Per payer specifications; otherwise leave empty.	Per payer specifications; otherwise leave empty.	Per payer specifications; otherwise leave empty.	Not required.

Block 24J—Reserved For Local Use   Purpose: Identifies the specific doctor that performed the services.

```
J
RENDERING
PROVIDER ID.
```

Information to Enter	Commercial/Private	Medicare	Medicaid	Workers' Compensation
Enter the non-NPI number in the shaded area of the field. Enter the NPI number in the unshaded area of the field.	Required.	Required.	Required.	Not required.

(continues on next page)

234

Block 25—Federal Tax I.D. Number — Purpose: Identifies the billing provider.

25. FEDERAL TAX I.D. NUMBER   SSN EIN ☐ ☐

Commercial/Private	Medicare	Medicaid	Workers' Compensation
Required.	Required.	Required.	Required.

Information to Enter

Enter the billing provider's federal tax identification number (include hyphen), social security, or employer identification number (include hyphen). Specify type of number by entering an X in the correct box. Use spaces to separate parts of field.

Block 26—Patient's Account Number — Purpose: Identifies the patient.

26. PATIENT'S ACCOUNT NO.

Commercial/Private	Medicare	Medicaid	Workers' Compensation
Required.	Required.	Required.	Required.

Information to Enter

Enter the patient's account number assigned by the billing provider.

Block 27—Accept Assignment? — Purpose: Indicates if the provider accepts assignment of Medicare benefits.

27. ACCEPT ASSIGNMENT? (For govt. claims, see back) ☐ YES ☐ NO

Commercial/Private	Medicare	Medicaid	Workers' Compensation
Required.	Required.	"Yes" box must be marked.	Not required.

Information to Enter

Enter an X in the correct box.

Block 28—Total Charge — Purpose: Informs the payer of the total dollars charged for the billed services.

28. TOTAL CHARGE $

Commercial/Private	Medicare	Medicaid	Workers' Compensation
Required.	Required.	Required.	Required.

Information to Enter

Enter the sum of the charges in column 24F [lines 1–6]. Use a space to divide the dollars and cents. Do not use dollar signs. Do not use commas as thousands marker.

(continues on next page)

Block 29—Amount Paid   Purpose: Indicates payments made by other payers or by the patient.

29. AMOUNT PAID

$

Information to Enter	Commercial/Private	Medicare	Medicaid	Workers' Compensation
Enter the amount the patient or other payers paid on covered services only. Use a space to divide the dollars and cents. Do not use dollar signs. Do not use commas as thousands marker.	Required.	Required.	Do not enter the Medicaid copayment amount.	Required.

Block 30—Balance Due   Purpose: Indicates the balance due to be paid to the provider of services.

30. BALANCE DUE

$

Information to Enter	Commercial/Private	Medicare	Medicaid	Workers' Compensation
Subtract block 29 from block 28 to arrive at the amount to be entered in this block.	Required.	Not required.	Enter the balance due if Medicaid is the secondary payer. Otherwise not required.	Required.

Block 31—Signature of Physician or Supplier Including Degrees or Credentials   Purpose: Identifies the provider of service(s) or supply(s).

31. SIGNATURE OF PHYSICIAN OR SUPPLIER
INCLUDING DEGREES OR CREDENTIALS
(I certify that the statements on the reverse
apply to this bill and are made a part thereof.)

SIGNED   DATE

Information to Enter	Commercial/Private	Medicare	Medicaid	Workers' Compensation
Enter the signature of the physician, supplier or representative with the degree, credentials, or title and the date signed. Use the eight-digit numeric date (MM DD CCYY).	Required.	Required.	Required.	Required.

(continues on next page)

235

Block 32—Name and Address of Facility Where Services Were Rendered   Purpose: Identifies where the service(s) were rendered or supplies provided.

32. SERVICE FACILITY LOCATION INFORMATION

a.   b.

NPI

Information to Enter	Commercial/Private	Medicare	Medicaid	Workers' Compensation
Enter the name and address, city, state, and zip code of the location where the services were rendered if other than box 33 or patient's home. Suppliers should enter the location where supplies were accepted. Do not use punctuation except "#" and "-." Use two-digit state code and, if available, nine-digit zip code. If block 18 is completed or block 20 contains an X in the "Yes" box enter name and address of facility here.	Required.	Required.	Required.	Required.

Block 33—Physician's Supplier's Billing Name, Address, Zip Code and Phone Number   Purpose: Identifies the billing provider.

33. BILLING PROVIDER INFO & PH# (   )

a.   b.

NPI

Information to Enter	Commercial/Private	Medicare	Medicaid	Workers' Compensation
Enter the billing provider's name, address, city, state, zip code, and telephone number. Enter the PIN, NPI, or Group Number. Do not use punctuation except "#" and "-." Use the two-digit state code and, if available, the nine-digit zip code.	Required.	Required.	Enter the provider's Medicaid number in the Group # field.	Required.

Index

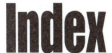

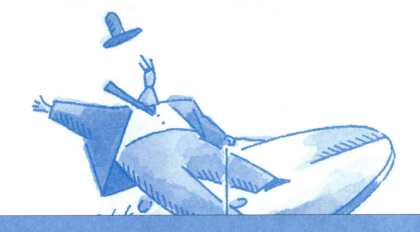